The Work of Play

The Work of Play

Child Psychotherapy in Contemporary Korea

Sheena Nahm, PhD

LEXINGTON BOOKS
Lanham • Boulder • New York • Toronto • Plymouth, UK

Published by Lexington Books
A wholly owned subsidiary of Rowman & Littlefield
4501 Forbes Boulevard, Suite 200, Lanham, Maryland 20706
www.rowman.com

10 Thornbury Road, Plymouth PL6 7PP, United Kingdom

Nahm, Sheena. "Between Stigma and Demand" Reproduced by permission of the Society for Applied Anthropology from Human Organization, vol. 68, no. 4. Winter 2009. pp. 406-414.

British Library Cataloguing in Publication Information Available

Library of Congress Cataloging-in-Publication Data

Nahm, Sheena, 1979-
The work of play : child psychotherapy in contemporary Korea / Sheena Nahm.
p. cm.
Includes bibliographical references and index.
ISBN 978-0-7391-8302-1 (cloth : alk. paper) -- ISBN 978-0-7391-8303-8 (electronic)
1. Child psychotherapy--Korea (South) 2. Play therapy--Korea (South) 3. Child psychopathology--Korea (South) I. Title.
RJ502.K6N34 2014
618.92'89140095195--dc23

2013042339

∞ ™ The paper used in this publication meets the minimum requirements of American National Standard for Information Sciences Permanence of Paper for Printed Library Materials, ANSI/NISO Z39.48-1992.

Printed in the United States of America

For my family

Contents

Acknowledgments

I would like to express my deep appreciation for my interlocutors. Thank you for taking time to share your lives with me. I begin with thanks for the interlocutors in this work, the therapists who shared their hopes and anxieties with me. But I would also like to express my gratitude for the interlocutors I have had the privilege to have in my professional and personal life. These include mentors and peers in anthropology, public health, community organizing, policy and advocacy, media and communication, education and family engagement.

I would also like to acknowledge Michael Montoya for constantly supporting this study, in its early phases of fieldwork, throughout dissertation writing, and in its final revisions as a book manuscript. Thank you for nurturing my development as a scholar and academic, and equally important, as a practitioner in the nonprofit sector. Thank you also to Bill Maurer for your feedback during the revision and writing of the dissertation, from which this book evolved.

I would also like to thank the Regents of the University of California and the Korea Foundation, for their generous financial support of this research.

And last but not least, thank you to my family (immediate and extended) and friends with whom I rarely "talk shop" because I cherish the fact they appreciate me for who I am rather than what I do. My work and play have been greatly improved because of their support and influence in my life. Thank you to my family (HYN, SSN, SN) for all your encouragement and support. Thank you to BN for being a source of comfort during the writing of this manuscript. To my friends and communities in Los Angeles, Philadelphia, Seoul and beyond: thank you for giving me a sense of community far deeper and greater than I could have planned for, hoped for, or earned on my own. SDG.

Chapter One

How Play Works

On a sunny spring day, long after the snow had melted but before the humidity of summer could envelop Seoul with its stifling density, I walked into the air-conditioned haven of a restaurant in a western corner of the city to have lunch with two play therapists. Both were relatively far along in their careers, but one was preparing to retire and the other just beginning to mentor others. The older of the two had been an advisor to the younger woman earlier on in her career. Sitting between them, my goal was to understand their livelihood as therapists and not to pretend as if I myself were a therapist. What quickly became evident was that the study of emergent therapeutic practices was part and parcel of the study of the contemporary socio-cultural fabric of South Korea (hereafter Korea).

Through participant-observation, a cornerstone method in cultural anthropology through which researchers pursue data collection through immersion, I was able to experience the daily conversations, quandaries, and adjustments professionals made as they provided therapeutic services to children and families. In many research paradigms, getting too close to the data is seen as a taboo and harmful to objectivity. For cultural anthropologists, closeness and familiarity is precisely what allows the ethnographer to capture the rich complexity of beliefs and practices through extended periods of field research. The admission of the "I" in the data collection process is part of what allows us to articulate social life as always experienced by human beings who are neither static thinkers nor devoid of subjectivity.

To complement participant-observation, I also conducted semi-structured interviews and archival analysis. This allowed data to be collected using a triple pronged approach, all of which located different kinds of data. My methodology revolved around the desire to collect data about everyday practices and conversations and see how they articulated broader social values.

Though the subject of this study was therapy, I myself was not trying to be a therapist or to write a manual telling therapists how to be or what to do. I wanted to bring the worlds of cultural anthropology and therapy together to see if new insights might be gleaned about the contemporary work and play of child therapists in Korea.

During the course of years of field research, I assisted therapists with sessions, sometimes setting up the room or sometimes being an aide to trained therapists during group activities. I held a camcorder in the corner to help them record sessions for supervisory feedback. I went to conferences with them, sitting alongside them during trainings and earning a few credits here and there in the process. Most of all, I sat and talked with them as they prepared and debriefed, reflecting on how hard the work of play truly was. I have tried to capture the complexity of their work and their play here in this ethnography, and tried to do so as plainly as possible so that concepts and insights might be intelligible to readers from a wide variety of disciplines.

Simplicity can disguise layers of complexity, though. This seemingly simple and specific story about play therapy in Korea contains lessons about the very messy convergences and divergences of stakeholders' narratives. Stakeholders included children, parents, teachers, and therapists; I chose to focus on therapists as the entry point for this complex story because they often serve as the bridge between individual and family scales and larger social systems. Initially, this study focused on a particular type of therapy and focused on the maintenance of a brand across borders. It became clear, though, that none of those questions about transnational program adaptation made any sense without talking about the broader conditions of possibility. The fact that programs could travel and land was itself indicative of a particular moment in Korea when child therapy was undergoing transformative shifts. At the heart of the narratives in this ethnography lies a deeper cultural exploration of the work of therapists who use play-based techniques to help children and their families. I trace how the therapists themselves constantly shape and re-shape their own identity as professionals and reflect on the challenges of studying emergent forms of knowledge and practice.

Though highly specific in nature, the narratives of these professionals also embodied the bridge between the local and the global. Not only did they physically travel through global networks to receive training and professional development, they also served as navigators balancing the need to retain fidelity to global brands of treatment models while responding to locally specific paradigms that required models and protocols to be adapted in order to be culturally intelligible and functional.

READING HISTORIES ACROSS SCALES

To understand why play therapy's story matters in Korea, why it matters in the context of the transnational circulation of therapies, and why it matters as a subject of anthropological inquiry, it is important to first deal with the matter of reading and reflecting on histories. The plural form appears here not only because history is always but one of many histories that exist and is shaped by forces and dynamics beyond the objective recording of fact, but also because histories exist as parallel (and sometimes interweaving) stories that are told across multiple scales. Individual micro narratives are articulated in ways that tap into diverse macro narratives about family, education, workforce, and wellness. Individual narratives collide with organizational and national narratives; meanwhile, locally specific issues converge (and diverge) with global flows of knowledge and practice.

Tracing scales is crucial to avoiding the pitfalls of oversimplified articulations of history, in its local and global articulations. Anna Tsing writes about the need to pay close attention to "ideologies of scale" or how entities articulate claims about the local, the regional, and the global (2000). This may sound somewhat abstract to listen in on how people articulate concepts like the local and the global but these narratives are often pragmatically grounded and anchored through concerns about supporting one's family (financially as a wage-earner and emotionally as a parent). Articulations of scale bridge the micro and the macro as therapists discuss their experiences with play therapy. These debates about scales come to life in the context of specific topics and case studies such as this one.

Paying attention to these various scales, let us return to the moment when I began conversing with two women that were major mobilizers within a specific network of play therapists. Recall that Dr. Yuh[1], the elder therapist, was near retirement after having established herself as the local "founder" of a specific style of play therapy. She had brought back this therapeutic knowledge after traveling to the United States and encountering a method of treating children that could be adapted for families in Korea. She returned to the local university setting and became a mentor to the first cohort of practitioners trained in this brand of therapy. Among this cohort was the younger therapist, Dr. Ahn, who was seated at the table alongside me, the curious anthropologist.

Dr. Yuh politely began our conversation by asking how Dr. Ahn was doing. Like many other middle-aged women in Seoul, Dr. Ahn was busy balancing work with the responsibilities of preparing two teenage children for an upcoming round of important school exams. These scores would determine whether or not they would gain entry into an upper tier college in Seoul—a process so competitive that it made me think Ivy League applications were a breeze. In a half joking, half concerned sigh of lament, Dr. Ahn responded that she was worried that her children were goofing off too much and playing too much instead of working. Dr. Yuh quickly responded, "Ah, but playing is a skill, too." The casual aside made my ears perk up with curiosity. And the phrase that Dr. Yuh, the matriarch of this therapeutic clan, used stuck with me.

This notion of "playing as a skill" began to be augmented and challenged through micro and macro narratives I encountered during my years conducting research for this book.[2] It also became a foil to another topic of conversation: the lack of jobs available for a growing and willing workforce. Many middle-aged men, who had once been ensured job security if they could just become salarymen at large corporations, were facing "forced early retirement." While the job market in Seoul had been highly competitive for many years, there had at least been some semblance of security with the logic usually articulated as, "If I get into a good college, then I will be hired at (insert name of one of the large corporations, preferably LG or Samsung). And that employment will last, as will my family's economic security, helping to pay for the educational services for my child to gain entry into said good college." But lately, these idealized pedestals of prosperity were being shattered. Those who wanted to work did not have the opportunity to do so.

Dr. Yuh summarized the times, again with her matter-of-fact tone, "If everyone plays, how will any of us live?" She vaulted from Dr. Ahn's individual laments as a mother overseeing the progress of two adolescent children into the conditions of modern society and the challenge of making a living in an ever-changing workforce. Dr. Yuh alluded to the idea that someone had to work to make a living and secure a certain quality of life for one's family. In a matter of minutes, she went from highlighting the importance of play as a skill (in other words, the critical work that goes into and comes out of play) to emphasizing the need for people to work to counterbalance a nation of growing players (by choice or by default by lack of job opportunities). All of these quips caught me off guard because Dr. Yuh was generally not a talkative person or a jokester. She was a rather serious woman who did not go out of her way to use puns or make ironic statements. For this reason, these two assertions about the need for skillful play and the need for workers in a modern economy anchored our lunch conversation. They became indicative of a cold hard truth emerging amongst professionals, parents, and youth in Korea: the duality of work and play as skills for contemporary life. Playing as a skill, tempered by the reality of wanting to make a living, articulated the basic work/play hybrid I found so intriguing about studying play therapists in Korea.

Lila Abu-Lughod defines the phrase, "ethnography of the particular," as a way of writing about "people going through life agonizing over decisions, making mistakes, trying to make themselves look good, enduring tragedies and personal losses, enjoying others, and finding moments of happiness"

(1991, 158). Ethnographies of the particular provide a way to write against culture, or to resist the temptation to totalize cultural phenomena—whether that "culture" is claimed as representative of "Korea" or "therapy" or "play"—while still remaining accountable to the thickest and richest description possible for events, people, and objects studied by anthropologists.

Writing an ethnography of the particular about an emerging group of practitioners in contemporary Korea requires an understanding of how things came to be and where they are headed without being bound to claims of rigid historical overdetermination. In explorations of continuous processes like program adaptation and emerging phenomena, it is helpful to ask two basic questions. How was the present produced? And what is the present producing (Falk Moore 1987, 727)? In this present moment, the work of play is being produced and worked on by individual, organizational, and national narratives—all of which are always-already local and global in nature. The work of play refers to what play does (what it produces) as well as what is required to make play happen (what produces it). To these ends, this ethnography is grounded in the contemporary realities of the therapeutic work needed to repair the inability to "play." These realities are articulated in different scales that converge and diverge to create moments of flow or friction.

NATIONAL NARRATIVES

I begin the discussion of the national narrative on play therapy not with a sweeping historical overview, but with a microcosmic moment. A poet might see the world in a grain of sand[3] but I saw a pivotal sociocultural question in a conversation several years ago in 2006.

I first met some of the therapists included in this ethnography during preliminary fieldwork in the summer of 2005 and followed up with them in the summer of 2006. By July 2006, I began to discuss this project with several professors in Seoul to receive feedback about how to further develop this research. I took a break from fieldwork, or so I thought at the time, to visit the air-conditioned buildings of Yonsei University, one of Korea's premiere private institutions. After knocking on the office door of a well-respected researcher of psychology, I introduced myself. My research project was somewhat interesting to this knowledgeable professor, but it was my past life in the biological and cognitive sciences that seemed to make him think I was kin. I presented my ideas to him and explained my interest in studying the adaptation and implementation of a play therapy program from the US to Korea. He nodded, paused, and finally interrupted (at first gently, and throughout the course of our meeting, more firmly) to suggest that I might be barking up the wrong proverbial tree. For him, play therapy was not really science nor was it really mental health. If I was truly interested in pediatric mental health issues, I ought to speak to the psychiatrists of Seoul's premiere hospitals. I responded respectfully by saying that I would reach out to those networks, but that my primary focus would remain on a small group of play therapists. Again, he suggested that this group might be interesting for researchers concerned with education, social welfare, or child development, but not right for me given my interest in the anthropology of medicine and science.

He explained, "Usually psychiatrists will set up their own centers to claim a specialty, and maybe then, they might hire psychotherapists. But a trained psychologist cannot really claim it's therapy; they have to say it's a rehabilitation or education program…Short term training doesn't mean anything really."

This prompted me to answer, "Ah, but this is why I think the play therapists are so interesting!" He responded, "But I don't know if they are mental health."

I nodded excitedly and said, "Exactly!"

He repeated, "No, but it might not be mental health."

"Precisely."

We went on like this for a few more minutes, in the frustrating but quasi-addictive rhythm of Abbott and Costello's "Who's on First?" To me, the fact that play therapy was not a foregone conclusion—that it was not yet "fact" enough in Korea to either be accepted or contested as such—made this group of professionals and their narratives all the more interesting. Play therapy was important to capture precisely because it was emergent and not established. It was still finding its way somewhere at the crossroads of education and mental health in Korea.

Studying emergent phenomena sometimes means getting asked "why" or resisting redirection to more established phenomena. It also means that there are no well-established national databases to tap into to calculate service referrals for play therapy. Despite these challenges, studying emergent phenomena is also thrilling. It means that trends change quickly and unexpectedly and in the case of studying therapeutic alternatives, one can trace public curiosity alongside individual interviews with practitioners. Play therapy as a type of psychotherapy for children grew in popularity throughout my research among practitioners and among parents who would enter clinics stating that they had seen this type of therapy online on a website, in a forum for mothers, or on a television documentary series.

A snapshot taken from the results of a Google Trends search shows the growth in inquiries about "play therapy" and "Korea." Searches have remained somewhat steady with spikes corresponding to periods when Korea appears in world current events. One plausible explanation for these spikes would be that the joined search terms are used among those who already have some interest in play therapy around the world but with more frequency when Korea surfaces as a place of interest in the mainstream news media. Because these searches are in English, one might assume that this trend graph more likely represents the search patterns of therapists in the US than in Korea. But upon closer examination, search volume is most highly represented within Korea, followed by several countries in Southeast Asia.

The results page for the keywords "play therapy" typed in Korean show a different and more powerful trend that can be compared with the English query results. These spikes are less about moments when Korea appears in the world news for popular culture or for conflict with its northern neighbor; instead they are more about curiosity surrounding this type of psychotherapy among Koreans. Interestingly, one early spike occurs right around the time that I heard of "first cohorts" formed after mentors went to trainings or conferences abroad, learned about various types of play therapy, and brought "it" (knowledge, attitudes, skills) back with them to their homeland. The spike subsides and a steadier stream appears in later years as practices are established and word spreads from family to family. Although there are ups and downs post 2010, it is clear that the volume still remains higher than the flatline prior to late 2005 and early 2006. Admittedly, the increase in searches after 2010 does not represent thousands and thousands of searches. But that is not the point of studying emergent phenomena. In this early phase of growth, as a new sector develops with its own workforce and codes of training and expertise, public familiarity also gains momentum.

These trends are not meant to replace data about service provision or referrals which more closely correlate with the growth of play therapy within Korea. However, public trends are important to examine because service provision or referral data tend to be incomplete due to the very fact that many services are provided outside of the medical system. Public data also illustrate the rising interest in play therapy as it relates to interest in Korean politics and international relations. This is an important aspect of understanding the national scale of the story of play therapy in Korea because it represents how the idea gains traction in the public imaginary.

Aside from basic trends and mental health statistics, data about play therapy services, referrals, centers, and practitioners are limited. Part of the challenge of conducting research about emergent phenomena is to concede that data will be elusive or ill-defined. Added to this challenge is the unique nature of services that establish themselves just outside of institutional tracking mechanisms. They may not be part of national databases which in and of themselves already represent underreported data when dealing with stigmatized issues such as mental health. Understanding these limitations is crucial to understanding this ethnography because it is precisely these limitations that call for anthropological methods that are attuned to different kinds of knowledge production that appear in a variety of scales.

If we look at the closest equivalent data, we see that even with underreporting and a great deal of cases and treatments being addressed outside of institutional tracking or national databases, there is indeed a notable increase. From 1990 to 2002 the number of mental hospitals in Korea jumped from 26 to 83, a 219% increase in a little over a decade (MOHW 2002) and according to the National Health Insurance Corporation, 1.87 million people underwent treatment for mental illness in 2006 (Kim 2008). Given that these numbers are conservative estimates, the increase in the recorded statistical data regarding services offered and patients treated highlights a shift from the past when mental health issues were not addressed at all in the public domain. Only a few decades ago, the family or the asylum were the two major domains charged with care of psychiatric patients in Korea (Park and Kim 2006).

Over time, mental health has become a growing public concern for both adults and children in Korea. In 1979, the U.N. announced the "Year of the Child" and shortly thereafter, medical hospitals in Korea began to develop specific pediatric programs. Prior to that, children who had psychiatric problems were treated the same as adults, without much attention to differences in the phases of cognitive and socio-emotional development across the human life span (Im et al. 2004). When specific pediatric programs were developed, much of the focus was on inpatient services for children with disabilities rather than a broader frame for understanding disorders and atypical development. Since then, outpatient programs have multiplied in both number and diversified in the types of treatments offered. And yet, nearly every interview (or even a casual conversation with a friend or family member) included pointed reminders about the specter of stigma around mental health and its impact on underreporting and hesitation to access services that could be linked to the heavy label of "mental health" or "mental illness."

One study demonstrates that a significant number of parents who suspected that their child might need care were not seeking out care, and that the disparity between perception and action was greater than that of other countries (Cho et al. 2007). The study in Korea aligned with results from other studies in East Asia and among Asian immigrants in the US who often chose less institutional forms of care when dealing with mental health issues due to cultural taboos (Kataoka et al. 2002, Prior et al. 2005).

Taboos around mental health in Korea are nothing new, and have dissipated considerably in urban centers like Seoul, but the effects of residual stigma continually surfaced as a major theme across the interviews I conducted. The one area where perceived need and actual utilization of services were proportional to one another was for attention problems such as ADHD. Researchers have suggested that this is due to the fact that Korea is currently a country where academic achievement is not only highly prized but where the environment is so competitive that small differences in performance could "make or break" one's chance for attending a reputable college. For instance, researchers in the Department of Psychiatry and Behavioral Sciences at Ajou University School of Medicine wrote:

> On the one hand, cultural value systems may have the opposite effect on particular types of problems, resulting in a greater likelihood that the parents may seek professional assistance. Whereas studies suggest that parents in western cultures were more likely to obtain services for children with externalizing problems, such as aggressive behavior and conduct behavior affecting others, the present study revealed that Korean children exhibiting attention problems were the most likely to receive treatment. With rising numbers of child psychiatrists in Korea, and a growing awareness of child mental health, attention deficit hyperactivity disorder (ADHD) has quickly become a celebrity topic in a country where a child's academic achievement is among the parents' paramount concerns. Far from avoiding the issue, parents are so eager to embrace the idea that referrals for ADHD have been overwhelming specialists across the country, which suggests that public opinion can be a powerful determinant in the decision of parents to seek the mental health care that their child requires (Cho et al. 2007, 285).

Underutilization due to stigma and overeager utilization due to the perceived benefits for academic performance create a *tenuous rise* in interest for psychotherapeutic alternatives. The researchers in this study at Ajou University go so far as to call ADHD a "celebrity topic" in child mental health as well as education. This juxtaposition between education and medicine, as well as all the peripheral issues involved in both topics, weighed heavily on the minds of the child psychotherapists. They wanted to increase awareness and provide treatment without inferring that they could produce a perfect child (or emphasize the shortcomings and imperfections of the parents). And yet, playing to that audience was often an important transition into either making the very notion of caring for psychological health socially acceptable or prompting a parent to bring their child in for examination of possible ADHD and eventually receiving treatment for an underlying issue such as depression.

As play therapy gained traction with parents, it became a part of the new "mental health story" within Korea. But this was not and is not a seamless absorption into a preset history. Instead, as interest in it grew, the very question of what is and is not "mental health" also expanded. Thus, the study of play therapy's emergence in a country like Korea is the study of any new form of expertise that appears somewhere in the borderlands of established or institutionalized expertise. This peripheral position posed simultaneous benefits and challenges. The institutional mental health story (and its history) itself provides hints as to why a new form of therapy would emerge in its borderlands. On the one hand, to be part of an institution is to receive support whether through insurance coverage or through respect from peers and patients. But on the other hand, to be part of that institution is to also be subsumed by its history of stigma, shame, and pain. The periphery allows emergent phenomena to test its relationship to established institutional history, thereby rewriting that history through its stretching and challenging of the border's line.

In the midst of the revision of the national mental health story, a rewriting of the education story was also occurring. Play therapy emerged at the intersection of these moving terrains. Along with other therapies such as art or music therapy, play therapy programs were often described to me as more popular among mothers and children precisely because they were fun and seemed less clinical. By being less clinical, these playful alternatives were less likely to be associated with stigma surrounding diagnosis and treatment for any mental health issues. When I explored this phenomenon further, some therapists noted that many parents who were offered a choice between these three playful types of psychotherapy would choose play therapy because it was *play* and could not me measured in skill level the way art or music could in art therapy or music therapy. In Korea's exceedingly competitive educational environment, children (and their parents) were concerned with not only attaining high scores in school and on standardized tests, but also receiving accolades based on extracurricular activities (cf. Park and Abelmann 2004; Anagnost 2004). These supplementary lessons ranged from sports like swimming or martial arts to music and art lessons. Play was one of the only domains of childhood that signified freedom and creativity, free from the pressure of rules and evaluation. (Ironically, evaluation of the ability to play and experience spontaneous joy through interaction was part of what brought children and families to therapists in the first place.)

This productive tension between mental health and education sectors were developing as play therapy was gaining popularity. This story of a new form of child psychotherapy shows how study of a specific emergent phenomena can be a concrete means of tracking scale-making projects that articulate new and old as well as local and global in national terms.

ORGANIZATIONAL NARRATIVES

Play therapists in Korea treat children with a variety of disorders, ranging from ADHD to depression, categories described in the *Diagnostic and Statistical Manual of Mental Disorders*, published by the American Psychiatric Association. Most of the therapists I worked with had been trained, at least partly, through workshops in countries outside of Korea. A small handful of practitioners were trained entirely in Korea, but even then, they had been greatly influenced by their supervisors and mentors who were part of the cadre of individuals who studied abroad.

The movement of therapists and therapists-to-be across national borders but within organizational boundaries makes organizational histories particularly relevant to understanding play therapy's emergence in Korea. When I use the term "organizational history" I include histories of entities larger than the individual practitioner, parent, or family but smaller than nations. Professional associations and training networks are of particular interest here because they serve as governing bodies and institutions for therapists who may need additional legitimization outside of governmental regulation. Some therapists in Korea have licenses maintained by the state, similar to clinical licenses in the US. But not all therapists practice as licensed clinical social workers or psychiatrists. In these cases, they need the additional legitimacy afforded by membership in professional organizations. They provide legitimacy to those establishing rules and quality assurance apart from national or state regulation. These groups are usually grounded in one nation in terms of its association headquarters but committed to sustaining flows and making connections at the international level. Organizational histories are "smaller" than national histories in their topical scope (the story of a particular brand of play therapy, for example, in comparison to the story of a nation). But they can also be "bigger" when they deal with transnational flows of knowledge and practice.

One such organization is the Association for Play Therapy (APT) which defines play therapy as "the systematic use of a theoretical model to establish an interpersonal process wherein trained therapists use the therapeutic powers of play to help clients prevent or resolve psychosocial difficulties and achieve optimal growth and development" (APT 2013, About Play Therapy-Overview). According to this definition, the variety of styles of play therapy available in Korea all fall within the general category of "play therapy." Within this category lie several specific "brands." While this ethnography is about the socio-cultural narratives around play-based therapies as they arrived and circulated in Korea and not on any specific brand, it is important to look at specific details embedded in particular case studies and organizational narratives to glean broader insights. For example, one service-marked brand could be considered a subtype rather than a different therapy altogether. In Korea, the therapists I interviewed were often careful to distinguish brands by using distinct Korean translations that reversed the order of words such as "play therapy" and "therapy play." Part of the differentiation came from the need for therapists to separate themselves from other competitors in an emerging market. It also seemed that they wanted to honor the organization that managed the brand and were invested in maintaining that branding as local champions for this particular modality. Furthermore, therapists trained in specific modalities also wanted to distinguish themselves from untrained or unlicensed individuals claiming to be play therapists. Play therapists can undergo rigorous training even if they are not committed to specific brands, but they do need to be associated with credible organizations. Locally credible organizations included institutions of higher education as well as various professional development associations. Each organization had unique styles of management that followed their own bylaws and governance protocols.

By examining the organizational histories of specific associations, it is possible to see convergences and divergences. I outline some basic milestones in two organizations, the APT and The Theraplay Institute, here because these narratives were made publicly available by the organizations themselves. They appear as the result of archival research rather than as data collected from individual interviews. It must be noted that these are simply two of many examples that illustrate the importance of reading across historical scales; they do not represent the whole of play therapy or play therapists in Korea (nor of this ethnography).

APT began in 1982 when psychologist Charles Schaefer recruited Kevin O'Connor to make his vision of a national organization of play therapists possible. Offices were located in Clovis, California. About a decade later, APT created the *International Journal of Play Therapy* with the hope of promoting and sharing research findings about the impact of play therapy around the world. A year later, in 1993, registered credentials were established (RPT for Registered Play Therapist and RPT-S for Registered Play Therapist-Supervisor) (APT 2013, Milestones). The Theraplay Institute began in the 1970s. Founder Ann Jernberg developed methods and approaches after her work in under-resourced urban areas of Chicago, Illinois and published the first book about Theraplay in 1979 (Theraplay Institute, 2013). The organization followed a similar path in terms of creating conferences for practitioners to attend and network, procedures for training, integration of research to provide evidence of effectiveness, and a credentialing process for trained therapists, supervisors, and trainers. Jernberg was one of the initial directors for APT during the 80s and to this day, many Theraplay practitioners publish in APT's international journal.

To understand how organizational histories became international, one must follow the people that moved across borders. In following the most micro of narratives, the individual's narrative, organizational histories link with national histories. The most micro narrative is actually a form of manifesting macro narratives. In this way, the individual, the organization, and the nation all move in parallel rhythms that, in a moment of intersection, create new histories that bridge the three and transform each.

INDIVIDUAL NARRATIVES

Although Theraplay was a creation of Dr. Ann Jernberg in the late 1960s, the program did not take root in Korea until the late 1990s. The program's circulation involves many networks of therapists around the world, and while the program is not well known outside of these specific professional circles, the tracing of the transnational flow tells the story of its American origins and Korean emergence. The point here is not to declare the program a worldwide phenomenon, or even a uniquely American or Korean one, but to examine individual origin stories embedded within that larger arc. Individual origin stories often get lost in the historical narratives produced by organizations and associations when in fact, it is often the idiosyncratic and sometimes serendipitous movement of specific individuals that facilitates the circulation of theories and practices from one place in the world to another. In those stories lie the emergence, movement, and reemergence of niche therapeutic markets.

Ann Jernberg was appointed as the Director of Psychological Services for Chicago's Head Start program in 1967. Members of this program were given the daunting task of identifying children who needed psychological services and referring them to treatment centers. However, they found that there were not nearly enough resources to meet the needs of the population. Based on her years of previous experience, she began to fashion a program that could train "paraprofessionals" to do the work. The methods she developed utilized play and were based in the theoretical contributions of Austin Des Lauriers and Viola Brody. Des Lauriers is most well-known for emphasizing rigorous interaction in the here and now during sessions. This was important in reframing the therapist-child relationship as interactive and intersubjective, rather than the therapist aiming to maintain critical distance or being the blank canvas against which the child would write their story. Furthermore, Des Lauriers moved away from psychoanalytical emphasis of the past or in fantasy, focusing instead on interactions in the present. This influenced the development of Theraplay because play no longer served as a metaphorical marker for the child's inner mind or as a key to unlocking past relationships. Instead, play could be considered a means of addressing relationships in the here and now.

Many paraprofessionals began by working in schools with students and by 1971, Jernberg and several other collaborators created The Theraplay Institute. The Institute was intended to be a non-profit training organization, and during the early years, focused on training local practitioners. By 1976, the Institute sought a service mark in order to "protect the integrity of Theraplay treatment and training around the world" (TI 2008). The service mark was one of the first indications that the Institute was expanding its scope to include more sites for the program. Because the Institute was a *training* nonprofit organization, the expansion did not involve a franchise-like methodology. Rather, they began to think of the possibilities of training professionals from other countries who would then implement the program in new locales. Perhaps the most major development, though, was the publication of *Theraplay: A New Treatment Using Structured Play for Problem Children and Their Families* in 1979. The publication of the book put many of the program's concepts and techniques into quasi-mass circulation. The book was later published in a second edition as *Theraplay: Helping Parents and Children Build Better Relationships Through Attachment-Based Play* (1999) by co-creator Phyllis Booth. After its initial publication in 1979, the book was translated into German, Finnish, and Japanese. Given the available translations of the book, it was not surprising that the program quickly spread throughout the US, Canada, Germany, and Finland.

Before tracing the movement of this program specifically to Korea and recalling the "new" origin story that began there, it may be useful to provide some quick insight into the background of the two co-creators and why their individual professional stories affected the implementation of Theraplay in Chicago. This will also provide a point of contrast for the entry of Theraplay into Seoul years later though a different figure. According to Theraplay publications, Phyllis Booth received her undergraduate degree with a major in music from Brigham Young University in 1947 and followed this with a master's degree in human development and clinical psychology from the University of Chicago in 1966. She then began to work in local hospitals, specifically psychiatric departments where she treated both children and adults. She eventually received licensing in marriage and family therapy, clinical professional counseling, and play therapy. In 1969-1970, she studied under John Bowlby and D.W. Winnicott in London as an associate at the Tavistock Clinic. She would return to London in 1992 to spend some time studying at the Anna Freud Centre.

Booth met Jernberg while they were both teachers at the University of Chicago Nursery School in the late 1940s and early 1950s. Together they began to develop a framework for the activities used in Theraplay. Before meeting Booth, Jernberg's personal and professional life took her on a transnational journey. Born in Germany, Jernberg moved to the US in 1939. She eventually earned degrees in liberal arts (1948) and a doctorate in human development (1960) from the University of Chicago. Like Booth, Jernberg began her career in clinical psychiatry. She also conducted research as an associate in the School of Social Service Administration, specifically studying emotionally disturbed preschoolers and their parents. After that, she worked as a senior staff psychologist at a local hospital. In 1967, Jernberg developed psychological services for the Head Start program in Chicago, before collaborating with Booth to create Theraplay and train local paraprofessionals. Most of these mini-biographical sketches are described in further detail in the preface to their co-authored book (2001).[4]

I summarize them here to highlight a few key points. First, the two women had ties across continents, in the US, England, and Germany. Couple this with the fact that they created a program based on the needs and resources of a highly specific population of children in Chicago. The roots of the program began with biological concepts about human development and local social context in mind, but even in its first urban Chicago iteration, Theraplay was always-already influenced by an understanding for variations across social groups. Second, both women had extensive training and experience in clinical psychiatry prior to developing a program that focused on the elements of therapeutic play. They also held markers of expertise that could be interpreted as forms of legitimacy apart from this new method/program/institute, through doctorate degrees from a top-tier university and licenses in specific types of therapy. Licensed professionals have graduate-level degrees and are subject to licensure laws, which often include a minimum number of supervised hours of experience and the passage of an exam such as the National Counselor Examination or a state-level equivalent. These requirements must be fulfilled in addition to attaining a degree from an accredited school. To practice as a licensed counselor is to make a claim to being regulated and accountable to these boards, departments, and laws. This is important to note, not only in illustrating the legitimacy that Booth and Jernberg held through these apparatuses before creating The Theraplay Institute but also because the US-based trainees I met at workshops had also received their licenses in therapy or clinical social work (or were in the process of doing so). Thus, their certification in this particular method of play therapy would function as markers of specialized expertise. Their training in this method was a supplementary way of gaining unique knowledge to a specific type of treatment, but did not replace many of their other qualifications to be practicing therapists.

While the program gained popularity in those countries and spread to a few more, only a few East Asia-based therapists were listed on the website's directory by 2005. Surprisingly, the East Asian therapists listed in the international directory on the Institute's website were from Korea. At the time when I began this project and looked up the international directory of therapists on the Institute's website, no Korean translation of the book existed. I knew for a fact that at least a few of the Korean therapists on the directory were not fluent enough in English to be reading the English version of the book as a sufficient alternative to a Korean one.

The next "origin" story is highly idiosyncratic, as was the first one, but it bears mentioning because it serves as an illustration of the so-called serendipity factor that so often influences the emergence of a new niche market. A professor who had already received her undergraduate and graduate degrees at well-known colleges in Korea happened to visit some colleagues in the

US. When she returned to Seoul, she began to incorporate many of the articles she had come across and skills she had acquired in her lectures. I interviewed Dr. Sohn, who was a student in one of these classes. I met her while she was in the final stages of obtaining her PhD. She noted how "in the beginning, we didn't give [it] that much thought, other than it being another type of therapy, one out of many. Music therapy, art therapy…There are a lot of types with a more specific focus." "When it first came to our school, when [our professor] went to Chicago University, she thought that we should do [it] in our country," she continued. I was struck by the replacement of a training institute in Chicago with an academic institution, and its miscommunication as part of an affiliation with "Chicago University."

The notion of "Chicago University" did not come from the Institute, and it is unclear who first switched out the name of the institution of training for an academic affiliation. While it is not uncommon for terms to morph in the course of circulation, particularly with new forms of knowledge and practice, the elision in this case is symptomatic of the symbolic value and social capital associated with various types of affiliation. For peripheral "expert" groups, networks and associations can be incredibly important, particularly if their scope is international. But when I asked one play therapist whether parents cared about her involvement in local or international associations, she said that it was not the primary concern. Instead, one of the first and most important questions parents ask her is, "Which school did you graduate from?" This core question and concern has a lot to do with the importance of college alumni networks in Korea. One's alma mater becomes a strong marker for professional and personal status. This marker often travels with a graduate years after they leave college, influencing prospects for employment and even marriage. I wondered if the therapists who did not graduate from top tier prestigious undergraduate institutions then needed the affiliation with international associations and networks to trump their local affiliations. Furthermore, I observed that even for the therapists that had graduated from top tier colleges in Korea, the association with the transnational and international associations was still important because it lent credibility to their specialized expertise. Social capital could be found in both the local prestige of a nationally ranked university as well as the affiliation to international, specifically Western, networks. This extra credibility could be leveraged by linking oneself to the roots of an association which had begun in the US several decades earlier. In terms of sheer numbers, this lent historical and geographical weight to the sustainability and success of the "new" program in Korea. The "origins" could be traced back longer, while the popularity, relevance, and efficacy could be cast broadly as global.

Some scholars (Amsden 1989, Matthews 1995) have suggested that Korea, along with several other Asian countries, exhibited a remarkable ability to industrialize at a rapid pace because they were "late innovators." Instead of reinventing the metaphorical wheel, Korea learned and refined Western technologies, institutions, and theories in order to benefit their own nation's growth (and be more relevant to their local context). Many universities and research institutions even hired faculty and staff, specifically searching for Koreans who had obtained degrees from the West or had already established their careers in the West. In business and technology, the main role of these "Western-trained brains has been to introduce and reprocess Western concepts and theories. . .and to legitimate with borrowed Western ideas what have already been put into effect by bureaucracy and business" (Chang 1998:221). While this may not be true for all businesses, the assertion is an important one to think with—and against. I say with, because the paradigm of late innovation helps to think through the larger context of knowledge and technologies that are linked to the West as a form of legitimacy. However, it is also important to think *against* the assumption that late innovators are necessarily just copycats implementing something already formulated in the West. Even in the circulation of a specific therapeutic modalities, there are *multiple* histories to be aware of, each affecting how the program lands and takes root and continues to move. These multiple origin stories in this case are important to consider together because they illustrate how the first origin story does not lead to a prefabricated product that is sealed off from the possibility and probability of new and different origin stories.

To think with and against this notion of late innovation highlights why there might be such an emphasis on association with international networks, particularly those in the West, and the specificity of the Korean context where therapists felt vulnerable to legitimacy claims because they were introducing new types of therapy that did not fall wholly in medical institutional paradigms. Because many of the play therapists are trained in graduate departments of child development and/or social welfare, they are not housed within "medicalized" associations and their relative hierarchies. To create their own form of legitimacy, they depended more heavily on participation in global networks. Some of the members of the network remained active participants over the years. Even for those who did not participate consistently over time, the appearance of such via affiliations and membership status proved to be a useful link. Rather than thinking of Koreans as necessarily always belated mimics of the US, I think of each as having its own particularities, in terms of the factors in its social ecology as well as the windows of spontaneity.

Once theories and practices "landed" in Korea, it was not enough to simply distribute and replicate. Therapists, who were at once apprentices (therapists in training for certification) and innovators, had to describe and articulate what services they were actually providing and how it differed from other services in the child mental health sector.

Korean therapists indicated that various types of therapy could be helpful and it really depended on what was right for the client. However, they emphasized that it would be better if two therapies were not run concurrently because it caused confusion. "I've worked with a child doing both at the same time…So the child got confused. So I told the mother to choose which she thought was better for her child, and I can't tell you which one to choose," recalled Dr. Tanaka, a young Japanese woman who had been studying and working in Korea for several years.[5] She was one of the therapists who highlighted the frustration of splits in her field between practitioners of specific modalities, when "really, they are both useful and it would be more helpful if the two groups 'joined hands' instead of creating a rivalry between the students of one professor and the students of another." The idea of "joining hands" is more than a friendly gesture, because collaboration between two local associations could benefit members by allowing them to network within a broader cluster of psychotherapists in Korea. However, at the time of fieldwork, efforts towards constructing an umbrella organization and structure of subsections within it were not their main focus. Rather, the priority was on each group raising awareness about their own type of therapy, expertise, and practice. The "umbrella" for the Korean practitioners came from the connections to international networks of colleagues as opposed to trying to gain entry into the networks of larger more established groups of mental health practitioner associations within Korea, bypassing local medical hierarchies for global circulation. This is not just late innovation and replication of Western ideologies, concepts, and practices. Instead, because local networks of psychotherapy and psychiatry are difficult to gain access to, play therapists must seek alternatives to facilitate their "home-grown" desires and innovations.

This ethnography begins with the presentation of three different scales of narratives: the national, the organizational, and the individual because definitions of play, work, and therapy all come to take on new meaning only when histories are read across scales. In the specific and sometimes mundane sounding realities of individual practitioner, broader social issues are found. Similarly, broader social shifts impact the everyday lived existence of individual children, parents, and practitioners. In the following chapters, I examine critical issues such as stigma, legitimacy, expertise, gender, translation and transnational flows. But in moving forward, it is important to underscore that each of these "big" issues should be read through the grounded specific reflections of my interlocutors as they grapple with understanding the work of play.

Chapter Two

Between Stigma and Demand

In much the same way that a multi-scale approach lends itself to understanding the complex layers that create a story about emergent phenomena, close attention to the convergence of seemingly disparate forces is also needed. Standing at the intersection of seemingly disparate forces like stigma and demand allows a careful observer to note moments of convergence and divergence, flow and friction.

During the course of my work with play therapists in Korea, many discussions revolved around the themes of stigma and social taboos as well as the increasing rates of depression and suicide. Stigma comes in many forms and focuses on many subjects. Sociologist Erving Goffman once wrote, "We and those who do not depart negatively from the particular expectations at issue I shall call the *normals*. . .By definition, of course, we believe that the person with a stigma is not quite human. On this assumption we exercise varieties of discrimination, through which we effectively, if often unthinkingly, reduce his life chances" (1986, 5).

This construction of "stigma-theory" is not always a conscious decision. Stigma can also be inherited from specific associations with the past. For example, modern psychiatry did not immediately take off even after it was introduced to Korea during Japanese occupation. Much of this has been attributed to Koreans managing illness privately or through other means such as shamanism or folk medicine (Chang and Kim 1973). The fact that this form of treatment was introduced during a colonial period may also have made people hesitant toward utilizing "modern psychiatry."

Contrast this private management of individuals suffering from psychological illness with the approaches following the Korean War. Shortly after the war, there was a spike of Korean physicians moving abroad for further education and experience; a significant number of that cohort specialized in psychiatry" (Chang and Kim 1973, 668). Many of these émigrés returned to Korea and began implementing these services. At this point psychiatry began to be established more noticeably relative to Korea's own past but also regionally more than other East Asian countries. Even in this small snippet of the history of modern psychiatry in Korea, it is clear that the concept of treating psychological distress in medical terms took shape over a long period of time, through the course of major transnational events ranging from colonial occupation to diasporic communities.

Prior to the development of a public welfare and national health insurance system, mental health was managed by the family. Personal preference such as choosing to treat illness with folk medicine played a role in keeping management a private family issue. Cost also played a role. For example, staying in a public hospital required money, and most families could not afford to pay for hospitalization. Even for wealthier families, going to the hospital was not a privilege. For example, treatments for schizophrenia often involved the use of tranquilizers or shock therapy (Chang and Kim 1973, 668). It was little wonder that diagnosis and treatment for any kind of mental illness was either hidden from the public or associated with stigma. There was not much hope in treatment, and the conditions of living themselves made these individuals abnormal and as Goffman would argue, inhuman by the standards of the so-called normals.

Skip ahead several decades to the wide array of services available in contemporary Seoul, ranging from psychiatry to psychotherapy. With availability and awareness, demand for practitioners to provide these types of treatments increases. However, stigma still lingers and while I refer to it often as residual or lingering, I do not mean to imply erasure. I use these terms to indicate change from the past and ties to the past. This makes stigma occur in different and more nuanced forms than it may have manifested decades ago, but not any less real. The nuances of residual stigma, coupled with new demands for well-being and healthy living, must thus be addressed with attention to the tentative growth of the psychotherapeutic sector.

The therapists I studied specialized primarily in working with children who had been diagnosed with cognitive and behavioral disorders, which sometimes included mild forms of depression. Cases also included problems with attachment and diagnoses more commonly known in the US such as ADHD and ODD (Oppositional Defiance Disorder). Autism did not come up often amongst the therapists I interviewed, although it was clear that there could be overlap between early intervention and mental health. The public discourse and research around autism is important and many other texts address its complexities in great detail. It is important to not confuse that discussion with the one here, particularly because I believe the stakes and implications are different—though equally important.

In early discussions, the word "attachment" seemed to alarm some autism advocates because they saw it as implying blame upon the parent (for creating a barrier to attachment and therefore at fault). The concern was understandable given the confusion and misconceptions around autism, and the stakes for parents and families who deal with these ideas. However, much of this concern around the use of attachment theory in play-based child therapy stems from misconception around attachment theory itself. The therapists I worked with were informed by attachment theory, as conceptualized by John Bowlby and Mary Ainsworth. *Attachment-based therapies* are simply therapies that are informed by these theories; they are more equivalent to therapies that are informed by other theories that explain phases of relationships and bonding in child development and should not to be confused with the more controversial discussion around *attachment therapy*.

While the types of cases, ages of children treated, and their families' socioeconomic backgrounds varied from district to district, day to day, and therapist to therapist, I found that my informants were tracing several key trends. I focus on these trends here for several reasons. Firstly, I did not have access to the details of each case that were protected by confidentiality. Secondly, these trends spoke of a contemporary present fraught with emerging tensions between lingering stigma and the demand for services that might enhance academic performance. The latter was more complex than merely making children studying-machines, as it was also caught up in the pressures of excelling in education as a way of securing social status.

This chapter explores the multiple and contingent factors that influence the growth of psychotherapeutic services for children and adolescents in Seoul. While major contributions have occurred in infrastructure, discourse, and availability of services in Korea, mental health and its related diagnoses and treatments remain a field that is still vulnerable to stigma. Even diminished levels of stigma in contemporary Korea contribute to hesitation on the part of parents in seeking treatment for their children. In this context, newer forms of child psychotherapy such as play therapy become attractive alternatives for counseling youth because they address issues in psychological health while also avoiding the stigma associated with clinical psychiatric settings. The growing interest in this alternative field of treatment and its emergence as a new service sector is thus produced by the convergence of stigma and demand.

RE-CONCEPTUALIZING CRITICAL PSYCHOLOGY

In the introduction to this ethnography, I outlined some of the recent changes in prevalence rates for psychological diagnoses, particularly among children. Part of what makes the specificity of child play therapy in Korea intriguing is its resonance with and against much of the critical theory regarding psychology as a form of power/knowledge. Building on the work of Michel Foucault, Nikolas Rose argues that the 'psy' disciplines in particular play a crucial role in how people come to understand subjectivity. The emergence of psychological expertise informs constructions of personhood and modes of self-governance as the 'psy' disciplines become a way of understanding who or what is deemed normal or abnormal in society. Rose's theoretical contributions provide a conceptual framework for understanding psychology as both influencing and influenced by society, emphasizing that critical psychology has often focused on "language and narrative" rather than "a complex of apparatuses, practices, machinations, and assemblages within which human being has been fabricated, and which presuppose and enjoin particular relations with ourselves" (1998, 10). This study explores the changing face of mental health treatment as illustrated (and contested) by discursive shifts in the 'psy' discipline and the politics of redesigning clinical spaces in Seoul. Language and narrative in public discourse and in private conversations with my informants were neither products nor precursors of broader social changes. Instead they were in and of themselves part of the complex and nuanced assemblage of contemporary therapeutic practice.

Perhaps the historical context of emerging disciplines and their role in social attitudes is most exemplified by Georges Canguilhem, a philosopher of science. In *The Normal and the Pathological*, Canguilhem traced the historical development of certain psychological and physiological states as categorically pathological (1991). Although his work influenced Michel Foucault and later critical theorists of psychology, Canguilhem's arguments were situated in highly specific cultural, social, and political contexts. Therefore, it is useful to think through his method and the issue of stigma and pathology in non-Western contexts without assuming that the conclusion will necessarily be the same. This is especially crucial in contexts like Korea, where the critique of psychology as a powerful and financially lucrative medical sector might be challenged due to the remaining issues of stigma.

In Seoul, the contemporary emergence of therapy and counseling for children is especially striking given the slow and fairly recent development of psychology in public discourse. This is not to say that "mental illness" or investigations into understanding the mind are anything new for Koreans, but rather, to highlight the sudden emergence of psychological services in society as available and possibly popular. Even as psychological services exponentially increase, hesitation lingers, and the industry is far from a booming socially acceptable sector of health care.

How people talk about and view spaces of illness in Korea is part of a broader story with local historical particularities as well as global inflections. The relationship between knowledge and power, particularly in clinical spaces, has been discussed at length in the social sciences. I revisit some of these arguments here because they highlight and fall short of explaining the tenuous reception of psychotherapeutic treatments for children in Korea. Many critical psychologists have built on Foucault's work by pointing out the power differential embedded in constructions of abnormality or pathology that label certain groups as social deviants (Fox and Prilleltensky 1997, Nightingale and Neilands 1997, Parker 1997). As powerful as the critical psychology movement was in addressing social exclusion and stigma associated with those deemed psychologically abnormal, the conceptual framework was not without flaw. Tanya Luhrmann writes, "Foucault did presume that madness had always existed, but he romanticized it in a way that, despite all his insights, did a terrible disservice to pain" (2008, 11). Luhrman reflects on the anti-psychiatric trend that emerged in the 1960s and 70s as an unintended consequence of critical psychology. She argues that this trend neglected the ways in which individuals and their loved ones suffer from mental illness and lack access to treatment. By *over-normalizing* pathology, particularly in environments where pathology is likely to be ignored or kept hidden, pain is less likely to be addressed. Conceptually, it is problematic to critique power/knowledge relations in areas where 'psy' has not yet become embedded in mainstream society. Pragmatically, resistant populations often under-utilize services due to stigma so an early emergence of critical psychology could be misapplied and perpetuate the tendency to ignore or avoid diagnosis and treatment. This can become particularly troubling in populations that have a history of resistance. I emphasize a *history* of resistance, because of the all too common slippage in characterizing certain populations as inherently resistant to psychology. Instead, I propose the framing issues of stigma with a more nuanced study of specific and contingent factors that shape attitudes.

It is also important to understand that psychology in Korea itself has been influenced by both Western and non-Western concepts and practices, neither of which are monolithic. By the mid 1950s, various models of psychology and psychiatry had developed in Korea through an amalgamation of domestic, regional, and international influences. The development of psychology and medicine in Korea has always been deeply tied into complex transnational relations. In the 17th century, Confucian scholars brought Western medical texts to Korea via Chinese translations. In the 19th century, strains of Western medical practices were introduced through Japanese military physicians and Western missionary physicians. From 1911 to 1940, missionary psychiatrists emphasized humanist approaches to psychology. From 1911 to 1945, Japanese military physicians and psychiatrists established practices based on biologic-oriented German descriptive psychiatry. Finally, from 1950 to 1953, a transition from Japanese/German psychology to "American dynamic psychobiological psychiatry" occurred (Rhi 1999). Thus, psychiatry "entered" Korea along with many other types of scientific concepts and practices and as an indirect consequence of these historical inter-national flows. But even then, psychiatry and other medical specialties posed problems of regulation and implementation within the private sphere because there was no public infrastructure to contain or regulate these services. Limitations to access and structural barriers combined with resistance to talking about mental health issues publicly continued to put pressure on the family as the main social unit for managing an individual's psychological health (Park and Kim 2006). Even after public institutions began to offer services, children and adolescents were given the same treatments as adults. This changed finally in 1980, when a surge of child-specific services emerged after the United Nations raised awareness through the 1979 "Year of the Child" program (Im et al. 2004).

The expansion and diversification of pediatric outpatient services for a broader range of diagnoses, from learning disorders to behavioral and emotional disorders, can be studied in a variety of ways. One crucial component of emerging mental health practices is the work of the practitioners and how they come into being. It is important to pay close attention to the experiences and articulations of the therapists themselves who are embedded in the dynamic shifts of their own discipline and practice that they are able to both reflect (and take for granted) some of the tensions in child psychotherapy. To this end, I now turn to the experiences and reflections of therapists who work in hospital settings as well as welfare, community, and counseling centers because they provide a wider view of the contemporary state of psychological health services in Korea. In their interviews, the therapists focus on the expansion of services and highlight the appeal of options like play-based psychotherapy that allow clients to seek treatments not associated with "institutionalization" or medication.

STIGMA, WHEN IT LINGERS

Stigma varies in degree and definition across populations as well as across bodies of research. For the purpose of this study, I refer to the assertion that "stigma exists when elements of labeling, stereotyping, separation, status loss, and discrimination occur together in a power situation that allows them" (Link and Phelan 2001, 377). A majority of therapists I spoke with agreed that stigma had declined significantly in recent years. In fact, they noted how some clients have not only become receptive to the idea of therapy for their child, but also taken their interest in therapy to a new level of hyper-consumerism. Dr. Kim, a certified play therapist who had been working in Korea for several years, highlighted the way sudden attentiveness to quality care has become demonstrative of consumer prowess:

> It's not just hospitals—pediatric psychiatric clinics—that are increasing. There are also centers that just do treatment. But if you observe, mothers, in the past (gasp), if you said, "We're going to the hospital" or we said "our child has a disorder" they would NOT like it. And going to the hospital? They'd think it was a crisis. . .Lately, now there are also many of these kinds of programs on TV. On SBS, "Our Child Has Changed." Children with problems and psychologists helping, these kinds of programs on EBS, how to raise children and tips for mothers and fathers. [1]
>
> If you watch on those channels, there are many scenes where they show people doing play therapy. So actually, those kinds of things also have influence on mothers. Especially if you see it on TV, instead of people feeling resistant, they're more accepting, so lately, mothers, like with buying things for kids: if someone over there does it, oh they're all interested. I've seen a lot of that. So going to counseling centers or hospitals, I think now, compared to in the past, it's less intimidating to the parents. So at childcare centers, if a teacher says, "Oh going might be good," then in the past, the mother would have said, immediately, "We're not going back to that childcare center anymore!" It would have turned out like that. Like, "That teacher is weird. I'm not sending my child." It would turn out like that. But lately, if you tell the mother something like that, they'll say, "Okay I understand," and of course there are mothers who don't go, but the number of mothers who will go has increased.

Dr. Kim's response illustrates how major shifts have occurred on both the provider and client sides of therapy. As an employee of a pediatric psychiatric clinic, Dr. Kim was familiar with the use of play during therapy sessions with children. She emphasized that play facilitates relationship-building skills, and is central to a child's healthy emotional and social development. This was a general statement about child development that I could imagine any number of the therapists I met at the international workshops in Chicago saying. But what struck me was the quick shift into what this belief and its related practice meant in the context of her own work environment. She began to reflect on the increase in places that provide psychotherapy, in part because people were becoming more open to such services. Dr. Kim, and many of the other therapists I would later interview, attributed a large part of this new "openness" to public education in the media, particularly television programs like "Our Child has Changed" on the popular television station Seoul Broadcasting System and online forums. Public perception has slowly begun to change and thus affected the changes in demand and supply of trained therapists in specialized fields like play therapy. More than a simple issue of supply and demand, though, Dr. Kim pointed out how psychological issues have been reformulated in the public imaginary. Popular television shows and other contemporary media outlets like newspapers and online fan forums that morphed into community forums where parents would share resources deeply influenced public awareness and discourse. Stigma still remains, she emphasized, but it has significantly decreased and made it possible for people like her to offer psychotherapeutic services to interested parents and their children. And yet, embedded within this hopeful narrative of changing public awareness of mental health issues, is a tangential but crucial tie to consumer culture, specifically the consumption of "quality" goods and services as markers of status and prowess in a competitive environment (Abelmann 2003, Nelson 2000). I emphasize the overlap between "openness" and consumer prowess less as a critique of capitalism (although that study and argument can easily be made as well) but as a way of noting how being subsumed in the rest of hyper-consumer culture (i.e., buying the hottest toys or sending one's child to the best tutoring programs) allows one to even be a *visible consumer* of a once stigmatized sector of service. Many therapists prefer to use the less stigmatized work "client" over "patient" as patients are often those found in hospital settings, rather than once a week meetings with a therapist. Furthermore, I use the term "consumer" here because the client is not only a receiver of therapy but also an active participant, who consumes the service, often through out-of-pocket expenditures. The slippage between openness to treatment and hyper-consumerism is not just an overlapping space that provides shelter from stigma. It is also a space where new issues and tensions arise, such as the pressure for therapists to differentiate their services and professional roles from other popularly consumed services such as educational consulting and tutoring.

I do not aim to set up educational institutions like hagwons [for-profit private educational institutes] and tutoring programs as a performance-based capitalistic foil to therapeutic service. Rather, I want to provide a more nuanced picture of the conditions that create demand for services for children. The hyper-consumerism and desire for academic excellence can too quickly be dismissed as another form of desire gone pathological, but it should be noted that there is much at stake in such endeavors. A study conducted at Hanseong Elementary School showed how educational settings like the classroom are sites of reproducing social status. Socioeconomic status influences the kinds of schools children attend, and their access to resources such as private tutoring after school. In the Hanseong study, researchers found a correlation between socioeconomic status and the expectations of teachers, such that the higher the socioeconomic status of the student the more the teacher expected excellence. This stratified expectation would then influence the level of attention that child received, creating an environment where socioeconomic status converted into academic achievement (Robinson 1994).[2] Add to this the fact that private tutoring for subjects like English add practical and symbolic value to children and their mothers, who often manage children's education (Park and Abelmann 2004).

Public demand for private tutoring, combined with increasingly fierce competition for acceptance into top-tier schools, has created an environment where academic achievement is desired at all costs and the financial burden shifts from the state to students and families (Seth 2002). In Seoul, most students learn English from an early age. Symbolically, mothers who are savvy in navigating public and private educational resources readily display their "cosmopolitan striving in a global order" (Park and Abelmann 2004). These displays of cosmopolitan and global citizenship, as well as basic displays of class status, are reproduced not only in the classroom, but also through the savvy of certain caretakers who bring their child to a therapist. Dr. Kim's interview suggests that it has become easier for her clients to be seen as consumers of therapeutic services, so much so that clients have become competitive with one another to attain the best possible services from well-known centers even if it means traveling across town for appointments.

On a slightly more pessimistic note, Dr. Ingram suggests that there could be another reason for parents coming from distant neighborhoods to receive treatment. Dr. Ingram is a therapist from North America who has been practicing in Korea for over a decade. I contacted him in the hopes of gaining insight about his own experiences with both Korean national and expatriate clients that he worked with in Seoul. He became an interesting source of information for those reasons, as well as for his insight into his network of Korean therapists who had become his friends and colleagues. According to Dr. Ingram, there were cases where parents were going the extra distance, literally and figuratively, to seek out popular or well-respected treatments, but there could be other factors in play. Although trained in North America, Dr. Ingram had been a counselor in Korea for a little over a decade. He recalled a particularly memorable experience with a colleague. Dr. Ingram had gone to visit the colleague for lunch. Upon arriving a few minutes early at the clinic, he was brought into a separate waiting room for several minutes. Dr. Ingram asked his colleague "what that was all about and he said it was because I couldn't see his clients."

"It's like that. At the Apgujeong-dong clinic, people aren't from the area. They go to Ilsan, Mok-dong, Jongno because they don't want their neighbors to see them. Clients from Mok-dong go somewhere else. If you're from Apgujeong-dong, you go—nowhere near Gangnam," lamented Dr. Ingram. "I mean, counseling is about *ridding shame*. A lot of Koreans are resistant to seeing a counselor." In his interview, Dr. Ingram used the various neighborhoods in and around Seoul to illustrate how clients navigate their way through clinics in order to find the best services *or* to maintain privacy. Apgujeong-dong is part of Gangnam District, slightly southeast of the city center. The other neighborhoods he listed are not in any district adjacent to Gangnam. In fact, Ilsan is outside of Seoul entirely, in a nearby province and district northwest of the city. Mok-dong is a neighborhood in Yongdungpo District, west of the city center, and Jongo is just north of City Hall in the center of Seoul but across the river from Gangnam. Here, Dr. Ingram is emphasizing the distance one will travel. In other interviews, reference to specific neighborhoods contrasted Gangnam (an affluent district, south of the Han River) with other parts of Seoul because Gangnam was the main area where therapists felt academic achievement might overlap with counseling services or where practitioners might be able to profit from their services.

Dr. Ingram also expressed deep frustration over the lengths people go to in order to keep their visits to a psychiatrist or therapist a secret from acquaintances. Even the more optimistic therapists who highlighted the increasing openness to seeking therapy were quick to agree that stigma was still very much a real concern. The juxtaposition of Dr. Jung's and Dr. Ingram's statements provides insight into the tentative rise of psychotherapy in contemporary Korean society, as psychotherapy has both benefited from stigma-reducing strategies and been subsumed under pre-existing proclivities like consumerism or stigma and shame.

RE-NAMING ILLNESS AND RE-MAKING CLINICAL SPACE

Because of lingering stigma in a growing service sector, minor differences in wording or phrasing have become crucial. In "Discourses of Illness, Meanings of Modernity: A Gendered Construction of Seonginbyeong," June J.H. Lee describes the co-incidental emphasis on sŏnginbyŏng and critiques of modernity in public discourse.[3] Seonginbyeong is a broad medical term that includes hypertension, diabetes, heart disease, liver disease, stomach ailments, chronic bronchitis, and some types of cancers (Lee 2002, 57). It would be tempting to label this as a culturally influenced medical phenomena or another culture-bound syndrome. On the one hand, it is a term that has resonance in Korea as a category for so many diagnoses. On the other hand, it is important to avoid suggesting that Seonginbyeong only exists in Korea or that it is conceptualized in this society in a particularly curious way due to a different kind of cultural construction and understanding of illness in Korea. All too quickly and easily, the logic could then essentialize this term as an example of Korea and its Otherness, and the Othering of its medical knowledge as someone confusing clearly separate categories in Western medicine. Instead of collecting samples of curious cultural constructions, Lee suggests that it might be far more productive to ask why specific biomedical manifestations are articulated in meaningful ways in a given moment in time (Lee 2002, 57). Instead of comparing Korea as an Eastern foil to the West, she examines the rise of this term in public discourse and its increasing prevalence as a physiological manifestation within the specific context of Korea at a moment in time. She asks not only "why here" but also "why now?" Thus, sŏnginbyŏng narratives emerge as an illustration of concerns about modernity and development's unintended consequences on economic opportunities for the middle class, family life, and individual health. The narratives of illness are then situated in the growing social anxieties of modernism and about modernism's toll on life and livelihood. The economic development of a nation and the work required of its citizens to enable this rise taxes the body, creating narratives of stress-related illnesses that become articulated in an illness that literally translates to "adult's disease," suggesting that any adult with responsibilities must endure these side effects and consequences of modernity.

A similar approach is useful in examining the seemingly sudden rise in psychological illnesses among children, as a fact to be noted by public health experts as well as an articulation of social life in contemporary Korea. This is why it is important to contextualize the individual narratives of therapists like Dr. Kim and Dr. Ingram with the broader popular medical discourse and its internal debates. The circulation of terms and their contestations serve as indicators of concerns from the private and public realms. For example, after Dr. Ingram emphasized the concept of shame, he suggested that one possible solution was to change the very language used to describe mental illness. One pediatric psychiatric clinic I conducted participant-observation at refrains from using the word "illness" entirely. Instead, it describes its services in terms of improving psychological health rather than attending to any abnormality in mental health.

The clinic's website states that it is "a clinic and research center that strives to develop character by harmonizing children's sensitivities and intellects" with "a unique program that works toward developing tranquility and efficiency of the mind. By reorganizing our lives and transforming ourselves in terms of these three points (behavior, thinking, and emotions), we can achieve true learning and the key to happiness." Elsewhere on the website, core aims are listed as: (1) "helping to know oneself more profoundly and nurture the maeum (mind/heart)'s ability;" (2) aiding "parents and children who are already healthy and seek an even more effective and beautiful life;" and (3) working "to further encourage/empower our friends who are already healthy, lovely, and full of potential." A critical perspective might suggest that the wording on this website is instrumental to broadening the possible client pool by making services attractive to "even healthy" people. After all, isn't nurturing happiness something everyone could always use a little more of? This may explain part of the careful choice (and avoidance) of certain words, but cynicism alone does not explain the discursive shifts. Discursive shifts are always more than a mere matter of semantics as they not only reflect the desire of practitioners to change the public's perception of their work, but also affect clients' actions. Later interviews with therapists, many of whom had no ties to this clinic in loyalty nor in financial profit, suggested that the wording was simply "making it okay" for clients to feel that coming to a center or clinic was no longer an admission of "crisis." By shifting away from clinical language toward the emphasis on self-improvement (while still providing information regarding the clinical qualifications of practitioners), this setting for play therapy allows parents and children to seek services without the anxiety of labeling their child as mentally *ill*. Thus, the promotion of this program allows for a softer, perhaps more gentle, mental health discourse.

Accounts of illness in the literature vary according to context and research participant. Medical anthropologist Arthur Kleinman examined cases of neurasthenia in China during the 1970s in *Social Origins of Distress and Disease* (1986). Kleinman observed symptoms resembling those of depression, as classified in the United States, but the patients identified themselves as experiencing physical dysfunctions of nerves rather than as emotional or psychological problems. This set a trend in cross-cultural psychology. Somaticization of psychological illness is now often emphasized in Asian American Psychology lectures for undergraduate students or to medical students who are taking workshops about cultural competency because a patient suffering from depression might present symptoms to a physician or emergency room doctor rather than to a therapist. Kleinman showed that these cases of neurasthenia were part of the fallout from the Cultural Revolution. Tanya Luhrmann asserts that the point is not to uncover the mystery of whether "Chinese neurasthenia is 'really' the same as American depression." She argues that it is always about a combination of factors like "genetic vulnerability, bodily stress, social milieu, cultural interpretation, family history, and individual temperament" (20) that are always entangled.

Lived experiences of illness, and how they are articulated, vary from context to context but there are similar themes that are common to most articulations. Estroff et al. focused their research on the issues presented by individuals with severe and persistent illness. Their "typology of illness" consists of the following: location (where the illness is situated); ingredients (what is unbalanced or affected); mechanisms (how the illness operates); and terminology (clinical terminology or spiritual terminology are two common examples) (1991). While many of the therapists I interviewed work with less severe and less persistent illnesses, their account of mental health followed similar typologies. One striking component in this research was the issue of "location" when describing mental illness in Korea. The word "maeum" doubled for either mind or heart (and sometimes both) depending on the context in which it was used. I translated this word in hybridized form as mind/heart in the transcription from the clinic website because it provides a glimpse of the duality of disorders the children are presenting. What began as a troublesome peculiarity in my early efforts at translating websites, brochures, and transcripts became symptomatic of the way in which "location" defied the Cartesian mind-body duality. This unclear distinction between psychological and physiological distress lent itself well to the growth of services that deal with both cognitive and emotional problems in children. However, it is also worth noting here because therapists would emphasize the "heart" aspect of healing relationships and the ability of children to relate and attach to their parents or peers. Meanwhile, the "mind" element creates a discourse where these services could be mistaken for treating cognitive issues and enhancing psychological health.

During my research, several reports of a beloved celebrity's sudden suicide emerged in the media. What followed was an intense discussion surrounding the problem of depression as an overlooked mental health issue in Korea. The media's spotlight on the issue can have vexed effects in that a sudden news blitz may occur after a major "event" such as a celebrity's suicide. While the blitz often brings much needed attention to the issue of depression and attitudes toward mental health, public education also comes at a cost. In these scenarios, the attention is sudden and dramatic, underscoring the "crisis" element of acknowledging issues like depression. Part of the everyday discourse of public websites and forums, then, is to circulate "softer" terms that make services about cultivating well-being and happiness as opposed to preventing crises.

Dr. Ingram's reflections on changing discourses and misunderstandings of mental health echoed the sentiments of a newspaper article in the *JoongAng Ilbo* published just months prior to my interview with him. The title of the article, "The illness that dares not speak its name," caught my eye and highlighted many of the themes from interviews as I read further. The article opened with a discussion of an internal debate among members of the Korean Association of Neuropsychiatric Practitioners (KANP), going on to state, "It's not just a question of names. Experts say that mental disorders are regarded as a cultural taboo because, traditionally, Koreans have believed that mental disorders are caused by demonic possession. The superstition still prevails in some rural areas where people often put more faith in shamans than in anti-depressants." Doctors had been discussing whether or not they should entirely remove the words "mental" from all the subfields that deal with psychological health for the past five years. This would call for renaming all "mental health departments" in hospitals and private clinics with new phrases such as "Mind Therapy," "Mental Stress Science," and "Medicine of Mind and Body." Psychological health itself is an example of biological and social elements. And in Korea, the mind-body split in dealing with health is even more blurred. While "mind" or "mental" was left in the proposed alternative phrases, the coupling power of "mental health" was erased.

Underlying this discussion over mere "naming" lies a profound worry that the phrase "mental health" creates a cultural bias that prevents patients from seeking treatment. Several therapists pointed out the increasing cases of depression among adults in Korea, and the article supports this claim with frightening statistics about the doubling of Korea's suicide rate from 2000 to 2007. Park Soo-mee writes, "In 2005, 12,047 Koreans took their own lives and 12.7 percent of people in their 40s say they have felt suicidal impulses. Suicide now kills more Koreans than car accidents or high blood pressure." This presents an interesting double-bind for advocates. If they emphasize the problem of mental health in Korean society, the topic becomes a "crisis" situation. A crisis then heightens fears about the stigma of admitting to a "severe" condition. However, if they downplay the impact, mental health remains a taboo topic that is under-resourced and underutilized. "For a long time mental disorders in Korea have carried a social stigma and psychiatrists try to reserve the phrase mental illness for more serious disorders like dementia," explained Lee Sang-min, a spokesman for the Korean Association of Neuropsychiatric Practitioners (Park 2007). The article and my interviews with therapists also highlight the *tentativeness* of attention and support for mental health services. Even as 'psy' enters the mainstream, it is emerging with trepidation and with stigma still hovering nearby.

The tension between residual stigma and the demand for more pediatric psychological services was echoed in many of the interviews. Another therapist, Dr. Chi, highlighted these changes in her profession throughout her own practice. A young woman in her early thirties, Dr. Chi had recently opened her own clinic after freelancing for several years. One major shift in her clientele was in the kinds of children that came to her. For example, ten years ago, she treated mostly "handicapped children" but now, "it's children with problems interacting with peers or problems adjusting to school, or difficulty managing their emotions." For her, the discursive shifts reflected the changes in her field. She later clarified that children with disabilities were still being treated, but often through hospitals and institutions where services were either funded through government programs or covered through health insurance. Because she worked primarily in private clinic settings, Dr. Chi was highlighting a change in the kinds of services people are willing to pay for out of their own pockets.

When asked if parents could now comfortably take their children to therapy, another therapist, Dr. Oh, replied, "Not quite yet. In terms of getting therapy, there's still concern that their child might be made fun of by other kids so it's phrased more like, we're going to a center or a research center. There are still many mothers who worry about stigma." Dr. Oh co-owned another clinic on the other side of town from Dr. Chi's center. She also specialized in play therapy. Dr. Oh added, "Of course, compared to in the past, it's much less, but there's still worry. It's not quite yet something easy to just chat about. Just recently, a mother told me that it was a big struggle to finally come here. So there's still some of that."

Dr. Chi reported similar experiences with residual stigma, but added that it was precisely this desire to seek help combined with the fear of residual stigma that prompted mothers to find therapists working in private clinics. "For people, the biggest concern is that the record of their child's visit will remain. So that's why they will purposely pay a lot of money and call a counseling center. There are a lot of mothers who don't want their child's visit to the hospital to stay on record because that could be a detriment to the child's future," she said. Dr. Chi then clarified that "detriment" could include anything from negative perceptions of the student from teachers, peers, or other adults to more direct forms of discrimination such as job recruitment or the lack thereof.

These fears are not entirely unfounded but they are sometimes exacerbated by fear. In either case, a barrier is erected between perception and behavior. The percentage of those who then seek out services is far less than the percentage of parents who are aware of information about psychological health and its related services. In one study conducted among parents of 3,477 children ages 8-13 in Korea, 10.4% of participating parents perceived a need for mental health services for their child. And yet, when it came to actually utilizing services to address their child's emotional or behavioral problems, only 1.9% of the participants reported acting upon their perceptions (Cho et al. 2007, Cho et al. 2008). It is possible that perception is over-representing the need for mental health services, but it does not explain why perceptive parents who could be viewed as *overly* worrisome would then *refrain* from utilizing services. If anything, utilization could help alleviate fears and assure the parents that the child does not need services. Or if services were deemed appropriate, treatment options could be pursued in a timely manner. Cost could be one deterrent, but fear of stigma also plays a large part in preventing parents from acting upon their perceived need for services.

To assuage fears, clinicians and advocates have resorted to strategies like "re-naming" as well as "re-making" spaces in these sectors. From visually re-making (literally making again) the lobbies of pediatric clinics and counseling centers to offering alternative treatments to drugs, psychotherapists and owners of these new settings pay careful attention to client perception. In my interview with Dr. Yoon, a young woman who had received certification recently as a child psychotherapist specializing in play therapy, I remarked that one of the pediatric psychiatric clinics looked particularly inviting. Dr. Yoon noted, "Hospitals can seem very sterile and harsh and so. . .you don't get that feeling there, because you can play," she replied. She was referring to a clinic that we had both visited, where the décor was striking in its opulence and lack of "hospital-ness." I had heard that an outside consultant had been brought in to provide suggestions for interior design, a practice I would think of as more common or appropriate for a ritzy café, art gallery, or architectural firm. "Red sofa, grand piano. That place is pretty well done. But from now on, hospitals are also going to try to do that too. It seemed like it was just at Child-Adolescent Mental Health Clinics but it's also dermatology clinics. Because you have to do the lounge interior well if people are going to come." The lobby of this particular clinic, in a wealthy area of Seoul, looks more like a children's art gallery or music hall. Parents can enjoy a cappuccino while waiting for their child to finish with therapy. Even the clinic's sign blends perfectly with the other businesses housed in that building: a restaurant, an alternative health clinic, and a hagwon providing tutoring services. The sign displays colorful letters spelling out the name of the clinic but not the actual word "clinic." So, for example, if this clinic were called "Sunshine Pediatric Psychiatric Clinic," the sign would cheerfully announce "Sunshine."

The remaking of psychological discourse is only part, then, of a broader shift in re-conceptualizing space and service in this emerging non-mental mental health sector. In a sense, the effect is just the opposite of the spaces created by buildings for the disenfranchised and pathological. In *Shelter Blues: Sanity and Selfhood among the Homeless*, Robert Dejarlais examines the Massachusetts State Service Center as a building that not only houses homeless people, many of whom are mentally ill, but also contains the everyday illustrations of the modern capitalist state's attitude toward the mentally ill (1997). The sterile and harsh architecture is demonstrative of both the problems within a state's promise to control and contain social problems and its failure to execute this plan, thereby creating a space where individuals are treated via medication and counseling but thrown out during the daytime. It simultaneously serves as a metaphor for the attempt to control via disciplinary power and the very lack of treatment to be found in such a place. In a space like this, the "culture of therapy is offset by the culture of capitalism" (1997, 177). Placing the description of the pediatric psychiatric clinic where many of the play therapists work alongside the mental image of this shelter for the mentally ill highlights several key points. Although the old institutions and mental asylums of Korea represent a different time and place than this center in Massachusetts, both serve as the harsh and sterile failures of state regulated institutions—against which private clinics now create their own space. These new spaces are still part of the culture of capitalism as it takes money garnered through the revenues of a private clinic to produce such a carefully crafted aesthetic so far from the old images of asylums. Creating a space that is like any other business in aesthetic sensibilities is oriented toward drawing in more clients; yet it has more at stake than just profit. There is still concern for people's feelings about being "consumers" of treatment for psychological disorders. By re-naming mental illness and remaking the space of the clinic to blend more with other services, practitioners are not only trying to diminish stigma but redefine the very thing it surrounds.

STIGMA AND STUDYING

Despite the fact that the Ministry of Health and Welfare has denied access to psychiatric records in the past, citing patient confidentiality, people are still concerned about their psychological histories becoming accessible to employers or the general public. In a survey conducted by KANP, 90% of sampled adults replied that they would hesitate before ever sending their child to see a psychiatrist. The survey results also showed that over 80% of respondents believed that psychiatric patients would suffer social bias and disadvantages at work (Park 2007). Given this aversion to psychiatric diagnoses and treatments, many people who suffer from "moderate" disorders that nonetheless deeply affect their quality of life are beginning to seek out non-clinical settings such as counseling centers or even using counseling services online or via telephone hotlines. Interestingly, therapists I interviewed who did not deal with more severe diagnoses associated with social stigma also noted fears of "marked" medical records among clients. These clients were actually glad that psychotherapy at non-hospitals (private clinics or counseling centers) was *not* covered under health insurance because it could be paid out-of-pocket, leaving medical records untarnished.

Some parents are also concerned about peers or teachers stigmatizing their children should they find out about their visits to therapy. Dr. Yoon also works with children using play in her psychotherapy sessions. She clarified that saying "center" was acceptable whereas "hospital" could be tricky. "Because the child might overhear, the mothers will say, 'It's a hagwon.' Or say 'we're going to tutoring class.' And in comparison to America, in Korea, hagwon culture is very developed," explains Dr. Yoon. "And many people study at a hagwon, so they can say, 'We're going to a class at a hagwon.'" This is particularly noteworthy as an alternative perspective to notes from earlier fieldwork, where critics suggested that play therapy might not be a "real" mental health service, and rather, "just another type of tutoring" for children. In Korea, education is certainly a plausible and powerful way of framing new services for children as exemplified in the earlier quote about hyper-consumerism. But here, a therapy session finds convenient cover in "hagwon culture" rather than necessarily being subsumed in the highly competitive cram school system. Thus clients are drawn to places where the name of the institute is less "medicalized" just as experts like the members of KANP generate alternative words for the services they provide (Park 2007).

Shin and Lukens argue that low utilization rates of mental health services are either due to lack of knowledge (clients do not know about services) or lack of culturally sensitive programs. For example, researchers have suggested that many Asian cultures, including Korean culture: (1) do not differentiate between psychological and physiological disorders; (2) associate psychological disorders with stigma and; (3) hesitate to seek help for such stigmatized illnesses outside of the home or family (Shin and Lukens 2002). I have hinted at some of these issues in the preceding analyses. Children's peer relationships are also affected by stigma associated with emotional or behavioral disorders. Social exclusion can lead to less participation in school activities, less engagement, or scholastic underachievement (Bagwell et al. 1998, Bush et al. 2001). One study analyzing data from 5,118 second and third grade students from 28 schools in Korea showed that the most frequently diagnosed disorders were ADHD, tic disorder, anxiety disorders, mental retardation, oppositional defiant disorder, and separation anxiety disorder (Yoo et al. 2005). Of these, ADHD was far more prevalent than any other diagnosis. This suggests that there are either higher frequencies of ADHD than other disorders among elementary school children or that the diagnosis is more likely to occur. Some critics might view this as over-diagnosis to profit off another prescription dependent person. But in this case, I argue that ADHD is simply more socially acceptable whereas people might hesitate to label children with other disorders, particularly those that carry more stigma.[4]

In a separate study of child stigmatization of depression and ADHD among various demographic groups in the US, researchers found that "the largest effects were found for Asian and Pacific Islanders (API) respondents who, in comparison with all of the other respondents, reported more negative attributions to a peer with depression and more negative family attitudes to a child with ADHD or depression" (Walker et al. 2008, 918). Furthermore, depression was associated with more stigma than ADHD. Although this study was conducted among API respondents living in the US, the themes represented by the therapists in Korea echo these concerns about stigma. Most available research in English focuses on the attitudes of Korean populations in America, focusing on levels of access among immigrant groups. While the experiences of Korean Americans are entirely different from that of Koreans living in Korea, I bring up this body of literature because of the embedded comparative analyses. In the research about Korean Americans lie several conceptualizations about Korean culture and the cultural barriers toward implementing psychological services. While API and Korean subjects cannot be clustered together simply because of ethnic category, I bring these two studies into one conversation because they both highlight the prevalence of disorders like ADHD, likely to be associated with affecting schoolwork and academic performance—and highlight the acceptability of diagnosing and treating such a disorder over other categories, such as depression.

While most of the therapists I interviewed in Seoul specialized in play therapy, one informant recommended that I speak with a former colleague of hers, Dr. Won, who could reflect on this subfield as well as her broader experience in other types of psychotherapy. A few days after I contacted her, Dr. Won and I met at a café and began to chat about her work at a major counseling center for youth located nearby. She told me about a few memorable experiences that illustrated the ways in which the demand for academic achievement is not merely driven by a hunger for performance but a broadening desire for children to develop "to their greatest potential" in all arenas. I asked if this then led to the question of whether emotional development is being appreciated in and of itself or because it could affect cognitive development. I was curious about this tension because many therapists had cited the growing number of parents bringing in younger children, who were not yet enrolled in schools, as evidence that people cared about play, attachment, emotion, and relationship-building skills in and of themselves. They insisted that they were not to be mistaken for tutors, or supplements to tutors. However, others stated that there were a few cases where the two collide—particularly when dealing with adolescents and youth in areas of the city known for the obsession over schools and hagwon attendance. One play therapist who was also a kindergarten principal, Dr. Eum, remarked woefully that the difference between children 10 to 20 years ago and children today was that "children today have more capabilities but the things they *feel* have declined, so children are becoming inconsiderate. They think a lot inside their heads, but feeling with their heart, emotion, or joy, there's not much of this kind of thing anymore." During our interview later, Dr. Won also emphasized this placement of "head" over "heart" by pointing to new trends in her field. She explained, "Something popular these days is 'learning psychotherapy' [*hagseub simni chiryo*] because there are a lot of people interested in cognition." Parents approach her colleagues with statements such as, "The mind seems okay but they aren't studying—maybe they need to receive therapy?" She then situated the main geographic site of this phenomenon and clarified, "But aside from Gangnam, to think that because a child can't study—that they have to go to a psychiatric clinic doesn't make any sense. But in the case of Gangnam, a lot of pediatric psychiatric clinics do learning psychotherapy."

At the time of this interview, I had not heard as much about the emergence of this specialized form of therapy, which focused on ways to improve the mind's ability to learn. I told Dr. Won that I was under the impression that something like learning psychotherapy would be more relevant for children with learning disorders. "Well, but if parents don't really know about those kinds of things, they bring them. . .But let's say they bring them for that, there are some situations in which they find out there is a more serious psychological problem," she replied. "They come for learning problems, but we find that there are a lot of bigger psychological problems. . .they come and we find out the child has depression. Of course, if the child is suffering from depression, the studying isn't going well!" Again, the therapists are presented with a double-bind. On the one hand, they want to promote the utilization of psychological services for children and avoid overemphasizing *only* learning abilities related to psychological health lest they be mistaken for another version of an already massive private sector of educational services. However, given the residual stigma surrounding issues like depression, it may be easier for parents to initiate treatment for more acceptable concerns such as difficulties in studying or learning if it serves as a "gentle" method of allowing for the diagnosis and treatment of problems such as depression. The elision and confusion sometimes provided shelter for parents who would rather say Child Center than Pediatric Hospital just as it would also provide the impetus for seeking treatment for one problem and ultimately attending to a deeper underlying issue. The sometimes antagonistic and sometimes collaborative relationship between stigma and demand was also a concern brought up during Dr. Chi's interview. She began by suggesting that "the parents who are preemptively anxious" about their children remaining competitive, being accepted into college, and finding a job often overemphasize the role of tutors.

Many individuals I interviewed were concerned about the overemphasis and frenzy surrounding academic achievement, sometimes at the expense of childhood playtime and emotional development. Dr. Chi suggested that some of the adolescents she treated were "tutored so much, they aren't able to study on their own. So during exams, if the tutor isn't around, they're really anxious and can't study. How do I study by myself?" Since her reflections resonated a great deal with Dr. Won's interview, I asked Dr. Chi what she thought of parents who might be overly anxious in bringing their child for counseling for the purpose of study, if it ultimately allowed them to be seen for potentially "hidden" issues such as depression. Her response added another layer to Dr. Won's reflections about the relationship between the drive and demand for achievement and the growing attempts to reduce stigma surrounding psychological health services. She stated:

> It's interesting because you see a lot of change in the first four weeks of treatment. Then from the fifth week, stuff starts to come out. Usually the mother is pleased at the improvement and right around the fourth week, will stop treatment because of all the time taken on therapy instead of studies. So then they'll stop treatment to return the focus to the studies. There are a lot of cases like this. . .So, it's common for us to just get calls when some big problem arises. And it's not like the child is a poor student. It's just that the mother is overly nervous. Later, I'll ask the child why he or she thinks they're getting that kind of pressure and it's because there isn't anyone else in the family who's gone to college, not the parents, and maybe not even among the relatives. . .So once the therapy seems to start working and they start adjusting better at school, it's back to the hagwon. Parents of teenagers, the careful ones, realize that it's not just about the studies but sometimes their relationships. And so there's a lot of change in that area too.

Although she was careful to point out there are many parents who are changing their approach and focusing on relationships and emotions in and of themselves, Dr. Chi's reflections and experiences emphasized that it is possible for counseling to be seen as a minor aid to tutoring—helpful in a child's studies, but lower on the priority list in comparison to test preparation. Taken alone, the reflections of Dr. Chi and Dr. Won provide great insight into the state of child psychotherapy in contemporary Korea, but placed alongside each other, they provide a more nuanced picture of the emerging sector. I want to draw attention to the juxtaposition formed when I consider Dr. Chi's reflections alongside those of Dr. Won, who emphasized the unintended benefit of overanxious parents taking their child for learning psychotherapy: becoming aware of their child's depression. Together, they highlight many of the themes traced across the interviews with therapists. The themes suggest that the residual stigma around mental health and the increasing demand for services facilitating academic achievement have reached an intersection that is neither wholly complementary nor contradictory. Instead, the meeting of the two has created a unique environment where alternative "friendly" therapies like play therapy can surge in popularity and interest.

The interviews and participant-observation conducted in Seoul suggested that being on the periphery of a system could actually be a positive factor for clients. This is especially true when that system is associated with stigma, as is the case with mental health services in institutions like psychiatric hospitals. Private counseling centers and psychotherapeutic services for children provide a more appealing alternative for those concerned with stigma. For some parents, the pressure to manage the children's health is part of managing their future, which should not be confused with solely seeking counseling for better academic achievement but is part of a growing pressure for parents to manage their child's chances for surviving and thriving in a competitive environment. Thus, spaces of slippage, overlap, elision, and confusion alternately provided convenient shelter from stigma and became subsumed by the rising demands overflowing from other more established sectors such as education.

On the provider side, therapists find themselves in a precarious position that was located at the intersection of residual stigma and growing demand. At times, they are considered to be outside the realm of "mental health" which can prove to be beneficial in assuaging fears and increasing utilization of services for children. However, being on the periphery also forces therapists to establish their legitimacy and expertise in other ways, such as through transnational networks and associations. The peripheral location of play therapy may also create another barrier for access. While it allows parents to utilize more freely services with less fear of stigma, it also limits access to those who can afford to pay out-of-pocket and stay off the record.

Author's Note

Portions of this chapter have been reproduced by permission of the Society for Applied Anthropology from *Human Organization* 68(4).

Chapter Three

Alternative Legitimacy

Play therapists in Korea often see clients who are less likely to be treated in hospital settings, both because of the family's hesitation to go to a hospital due to stigma around clinical care and because these cases are thought of as "too mild" for clinical care. In this "mild to moderate" range, parents notice a need for their children to receive help but do not think the cases are acute emergencies warranting inpatient care or prescription medication. In short, parents and children find themselves in need of services somewhere on the periphery of mental health.

In order to better understand how the inside and outside of child mental health services is defined, I began to interview hospital administrators, private clinic owners who were themselves medical doctors or therapists, and policy experts. There was some confusion as to whether play therapy could be covered under insurance with one interlocutor stating that it could while the rest insisted that it could not. This confusion was symptomatic of a sector growing faster than statistical databases could track. If play therapy was a portal to better understanding how child mental health was being renegotiated, it was important to examine key milestones in the development of policies and institutions defining mental health.

The Korean health care system has been described as "a privatized model with decentralized administration and fragmented governmental responsibility" (Flynn and Chung 1990, 238). During the time of fieldwork, the World Health Organization (WHO) reported on the state of the mental health system in Korea, outlining rates of service utilization and addressing mental health legislation in 2004 and revisions to national mental health policy in 2006. Policy change included: organization of services, human resources, access, advocacy and promotion, financing, monitoring, quality improvement, and accreditation. According to the WHO, there are 1,031 outpatient mental health facilities in Korea; only 5% are designated for children and adolescents (2006, 9). Day treatment facilities and community-based facilities also show low rates of child-specific units, and low percentages of children or adolescents among those utilizing these facilities.

WHO data also show that children or adolescent units were miniscule and that in general, patients treated in mental health facilities were largely diagnosed with schizophrenia (67% of patients at mental hospitals and 47% at inpatient units) or neurotic disorders (44% of patients at outpatient facilities). These were the most common diagnoses at the three types of facilities (2006, 15). For parents of children suffering from a wide variety of psychosocial issues, the need to do something was great but not one that could be met by mainstream medical institutions. Faced with this predicament, parents began to seek out alternative solutions and through this new "client" pool, play therapists began to make a living and redefine livelihood, both for themselves and for children who could access services without "being institutionalized". This chapter examines how therapeutic practices positioned outside of, or on the periphery of, governmental regulation found alternate forms of legitimacy. But before looking at the rise of alternate (and as I will argue, transnational) forms of legitimacy, it is important to understand just how mental health policy developed in Korea and how its evolutionary trajectory shaped burgeoning practices.

INSIDE AND OUTSIDE OF UNIVERSAL COVERAGE

Korea's mental health policy developed in the midst of dramatic economic development. For this reason, scholars of mental health policy often describe it as an example of the "productivist welfare capitalism thesis" which describes social policy as an instrument of, and subordinate to, economic growth (Esping-Anderson 1990, Holliday 2000, Kwon and Holliday 2007). Because of the ups and downs of democratization and because of the surges in economic development that occurred within the span of just a few decades, Korea is often described as an example of rapid political, economic, and social change (Armstrong 2002). As Korean economic development began to accelerate, the government initiated several large-scale projects. For example, during its fourth consecutive 5-Year Economic Development Plans, the Korean government began to implement a national health care system.[1] In July 1977, compulsory coverage for companies with over 500 employees was established. Former Assistant Secretary for Planning and Evaluation at the U.S. Department of Health and Human Services Gerard F. Anderson writes, "At that time, less than 10 percent of the population had any health insurance, and the per capita income was less than $800. Although Korea has experienced considerable political turmoil in the intervening years, it achieved its goal of universal health insurance coverage one year early" (Anderson 1989, 25). Coverage for employees was extended incrementally after 1977 by dividing the population into categories of employment and residence (companies with over 100 employees by January 1981; rural self-employed individuals and companies with more than 5 employees in January 1988; and self-employed individuals in urban areas by January 1989). In 12 short years, Korea went from virtually no health care infrastructure to universal coverage (NHIC 2001).

One way of interpreting the early categorization of health care based on labor and employment is that the government deemed the health of its labor force, particularly those involved in manufacturing, as a key building block of rapid industrialization (Flynn and Chung 1990, 242). During my conversations with Dr. Kang, a leading public health expert at a top university in Seoul who spent years working for the Asian branch of the WHO and as a consultant for the Korean National Health Insurance Corporation (NHIC), I heard an alternate perspective: health insurance was an act of political legitimization during the Park Chung Hee era. "There was rapid economic development, but also political oppression of democratic movements, so there was no legitimacy. Instead of political democracy, he wanted to demonstrate some kind of social plan. So, that was the start." Dr. Kang continues, "Health policy is often seen as a kind of social welfare policy but it was not really a welfare policy to target the poor in this case. Not just a welfare issue, but a labor/market policy: an *economic* policy. So, we can think of health policy as a tool of economic policy, subordinate to labor/market policy." Dr. Kang refers to the productivist welfare capitalism thesis here to explain how health insurance began as a way to assuage workers protesting against of an authoritarian regime. Whether the benevolent preservation of the health of a nation's labor force *or* the bargaining chip of a government willing to repress rights for the sake of development—it is clear that health care policy was inextricably tangled up in Korea's national narrative of economic development. From workers and their dependents, health insurance sprang forth to cover the entire citizenry.

This surge in policy and infrastructure was contingent upon several factors that highlight the juxtaposition of private and public domains in Korean health care. First, implementation of a new policy began under authoritarian leadership. The majority of this 12-year period of health care expansion occurred under the authoritarian regimes of Park Chung Hee (1963-1979) and Chun Doo Hwan (1980-1988). It was unusual for a country to attempt this grand a structural overhaul in health care at such an early stage of economic development. Anderson suggests that citizens had "a higher income elasticity for health care services than most other countries" because Koreans ranked health as the most important issue affecting their lives and the one most closely associated with happiness in Gallup polls (27). Thus, even in the context of authoritarian governance, cultural factors (and the beliefs of citizens) contributed to conditions that made universal health care a priority for the nation.

This idea of health as a social priority was echoed in 2004. David Scofield writes, "Well-being, a phrase brimming with marketing value, is everywhere in Korea these days. Restaurants, pharmacies, health clubs—virtually every service available in the country is prefacing the service on offer with 'well-being.' But while the term resonates with some people, exactly how all this wellness is to be achieved is less apparent" (Scofield 2004). While this high value on health is still the case in contemporary Korea, especially in recent "well-being" campaigns, it is also important to acknowledge its earlier form during the years of authoritarian rule. Government expanded health care as a means to economic development (to ensure productivity of a healthy workforce) but the cultural support for health as a priority to the nation also played a role.

Second, universal coverage was made possible through a partnership, if not dependent relationship, with the private sector. The rapid implementation of health care depended on larger companies to provide coverage to their employees through "medical insurance societies." For this reason, this system is often described as one of the few universal systems to rely so heavily on the private sector with the government taking the proverbial back seat. This was an example of both government and business playing significant roles in the evolution of this system, as did the individual citizen who continued to contribute to the system through tax as well as co-pay for services. Dependence on the private sector, however, hardly implies absence of government especially in the context of authoritarian leadership and bureaucratic management in the initial stages of development. Fittingly, the most significant movement in reforming this original compulsory system came from President Kim Dae Jung, a political dissident during the Park and Chun regimes who later played an integral role in including civic groups during the reform process (Kwon and Reich 2005). Ultimately, physicians mobilized and had more power in terms of renegotiating the deals of the reform and restricting the scope of the new policies (Kwon 2003). The lobbying power of the Korea Medical Association, "like that of its counterpart in the United States, enjoys a powerful position and has actively discouraged alternative forms of health care provision, such as new roles for paraprofessionals" (Flynn and Chung 1990, 242).

Medical insurance societies were formed to collect revenues, determine benefits, and accumulate reserves. For-profit corporations often owned medical insurance societies as subsidiaries that did not earn profit based on their activities (Anderson 26). To supplement the management of health care by these societies, the government also implemented a medical aid program to cover indigent populations characterized as: individuals living in public facilities, unemployed individuals who depend on family for financial assistance; and/or those eligible due to high medical expenses. During the period of implementation (1977-1989), government-funded medical aid covered roughly 10% of the population.

While medical insurance societies were charged with regulating coverage, the private sector grew more and more involved in health care management. Before health care reform in 1999, health insurance societies served specific parts of the population classified according to employment status and place of residence. Three types of societies existed. The first category included 142 societies who managed industrial workers and their dependents; the second was for employees of the public sector such as government employees and teachers; and the third included 227 health insurance groups for the self-employed, further classified by urban or rural residence (Kwon & Reich). Because their services were assigned so specifically, these societies did not compete with one other.

However, there was a different kind of challenge. Concerns over inequity such as the discrepancies in rates of contribution for similar benefits grew so medical insurance societies became integrated into a single-payer system under the NHIC. However, this consolidation under the government did not eliminate the role of the private sector.

For example, today, approximately 90% of hospitals in Korea are privately owned, often by physicians who are practitioners as well as entrepreneurs (Kwon and Reich). Medical care continues to occupy the intersection of private entrepreneurship, political management, and service. The extent to which each is emphasized depends on the individual practitioner's affiliations and personal/professional commitments. Korea does not fall easily into a public or private sector management model, nor does it align easily with the notion of health care as a commodity in a free market capitalistic system or as a right for all in a socialized system.

Government leaders chose to include health care management in their later efforts to stimulate the industrialization of Korea and interject the country within a global market.[2] In these efforts and their partnership with business conglomerates to accomplish such a goal, "market intervention" takes on an entirely different resonance. As health care management moved from the private sphere to the public sphere, it also fell squarely in the intersection between the private and public sectors.

Dr. Roh is Dean of a School of Medicine in Korea. Like Dr. Kang, Dr. Roh had worked with both the Ministry of Health and Welfare (MOHW) and the NHIC prior to entering academia. He sat down with me over a meal and explained the difference between governmental and market forces on Korea's health care system. He explained that a specific budget for health care is set aside from citizens' contributions. The head of the MOHW then determines the amount of the contribution that goes toward that budget. Because it was difficult for the government to deal with all of the management issues involved in health care, officials set up the NHIC to keep things organized. One of the main critiques leveled against this process has been the lack of access for citizens to provide input into the decisions made within this system. Dr. Roh explains, "Usually, the owner is the person who pays right? So the representative should be chosen by the people [because the people are paying], but in actuality, the head is appointed by the government. The president chooses the head. [The government's contribution] is about 10% of the NHIC budget, but the level of government involvement is more indicative of a 40% contribution." He also explained that when a hospital opens, it must register with the MOHW, and the hospital must receive 100% of all insured patients. They then charge patients using a fixed price list set by the government.

Elements of arguments used by both proponents and opponents of universal health care could be found within Dr. Roh's explanation. The assurance of receiving all patients compels those who believe in health as a universal human right, and not a product or service to be purchased in a market economy. However, the lack of transparency and choice is worrisome to opponents who would have issues with the government appointing managers of a budget composed of citizens' contributions. Price fixing in and of itself is a subtopic that can lead to fiery debates about the advantages of regulating costs for medical services, namely that it can either make services more accessible and affordable or that it can lead to mediocrity in providing quality service. This subtopic alone could fill an entirely separate and lengthy book. What I want to highlight here is the idea that even with universal coverage, the Korean system still leaves room for co-paying for services and full payment for non-covered services. That is to say, the development of a universal health care system that included mental health legislation and policy created important ways of tracking utilization data and monitoring quality of services but this system did not include *all* services.

Dr. Kang continued to expand on a key point in understanding mental health services within the broader policy story. "Universal coverage means universal coverage of the population but it does not mean universal services—so we have to figure out which services to cover first." He continued, "There are different approaches to answering this question. One is according to cost effectiveness and the other is by cost (i.e., more expensive technological innovations and more technical procedures)." Dr. Kang described how the government's approach to answering this fundamental question had been "an ad hoc patchwork style of developing health policy."

Not all services are covered and those that are often require co-pay. Dr. Roh continues, "About 50% is covered by insurance. The three main things *not* covered by insurance are (1) Food, for in-patient stays, but lately that's also covered about 50%, (2) Specialty procedures, and (3) When you're admitted, the amount of people per room that can be covered, depending on what level of coverage you have, is set. And if your insurance covers a room that is for six people to share, but all of those types of rooms are taken, then you have to pay out-of-pocket for a more private room. These are the three main things, but generally, the other examinations are covered." This non-universality of covered services keeps over-utilization rates down, but also has unintended effects in the service-seeking behaviors of clients for non-insured treatments.

Dr. Sohn, who I introduced earlier as she explained the relationship between therapist and clinic owners in a new market, also had much to say about services that are not covered by insurance and require out-of-pocket payments. She explained that, because play therapy is not covered by insurance, she receives anywhere between 50-80,000 won per session (roughly between $30-60 in US currency). Including the overhead that goes to the hospital's income, this means that clients are often paying much more than that. "Because it's not [covered by insurance], for 50 minutes, I receive 50-80,000 won. So for a mother, that's like 2,000,000 won a month at the very least. In Korea, insurance covers when you prescribe meds. Because it's medical, you can get it covered by health insurance. But it's not like that for play therapy or art therapy," she said, adding, "Those are optional and they're not covered. So for people who don't have money, they go to welfare centers and at the welfare center, wait two to three years." "Going to welfare centers" was a reference to specific play therapy sites in family resource centers, oftentimes located across from government subsidized apartment complexes, but it was also a reference to clients seeking services in centers outside of the medical complex. Other therapists echoed the problem of long waiting lists at public centers. Care, though accessible to all under universal health care, seemed to still stratify services inside and outside of its system—both by influencing the therapists being drawn to work in certain settings over others and by the places that are accessible to families who can or cannot afford out-of-pocket expenses such as a child's therapy.

The therapists I interviewed were not paid extravagant amounts, neither by my outsider American perspective nor by Korean perspective when thinking about the cost of living in Seoul. A larger percentage of what was collected seemed to go directly to the therapists in public centers than in private clinics which charged exponentially more per session but kept a larger percentage to cover overhead costs (such as monthly leases for space) and the salaries of administrators.

Clients, as well as patients for other medical services, in Korea are savvier than people might assume in a "universal" system, as Dr. Roh noted. They often ask other people or conduct searches online in order to determine the places they can be assured of receiving a certain quality of care. While Dr. Roh mentioned that when prices are fixed, people will go to more institutionalized or regulated places such as large university hospitals for assurance of care, the strategies may differ for therapies that are not covered by insurance and thereby unregulated in cost. Clients who could afford to do so, would search for the best quality clinics, centers, or wings of hospitals. Some of the most reputable ones were often indicated by the price of the session and the location of the center in areas of the city associated with "quality" for children's services.

Ironically, many of the therapists I interviewed worked in both public and private settings, and were essentially conducting the same sessions at an expensive clinic in a ritzy part of town as they were in a welfare center on the opposite side of the city. The issues of each client differed as they do on the basis of each unique individual's needs as did the needs of the families involved, which could vary on a more systematic level such as by socioeconomic class and neighborhood of residence. The structural and social environments among client populations differed in such a way that the child's interaction with parents, child's educational opportunities, neighborhood environment, and parental pressures contrasted. For example, parents were more likely to be "involved" in planning and scheduling their children's academic and extracurricular development. This could mean that they were more attentive to the need for therapy, or conversely, that they might be overly preoccupied with either the utility of therapy for the sake of improving learning ability or highly demanding of the therapists to churn out results in much the same way a tutor would be evaluated on his or her student's change in performance. At the same time, these parents are also most likely to be able to afford and seek out the best—the best tutoring programs and the most qualified therapists. Money aside, these circles are often the most well informed and densely connected where information and advice is readily exchanged with one another. This is not simply a matter of the poor going to local centers and the rich going to private clinics. For example, the wealthier the client the more they may want to maintain a level of status for their child and their families, free from any potential stigma like the kind associated with receiving treatment for psychological issues. Furthermore, the public center is not always the lesser of the two in terms of quality. As I have already mentioned, the freelance therapists often circulate in between these settings, sometimes during the course of a single day.

Additionally, the non-hospital setting has its own allure and assurance of confidentiality. While welfare and community centers were generally cheaper and more likely to be utilized by lower income families, I noticed that there were also a lot of middle-income families that could go either way depending on cost. The private clinics themselves often chose to be called "centers" rather than hospitals due to the stigma of going to any institutional setting related to psychological issues or mental health. This is counterintuitive to the assumption that the large university hospital symbolizes higher quality care or regulated services in comparison to independently run counseling centers. Herein lies a critical difference from the way "medically covered" services play out in influencing service-seeking behaviors and the way clients respond to finding quality services that are on the periphery of institutional regulation.

One could argue that non-affluent families are left with only unfavorable stigmatized settings like public hospitals or the welfare centers offered only to lower socioeconomic families. But there is another factor in play. One therapist noted, "Of course, there's a big difference with welfare centers but between counseling centers and hospitals, it's almost the same. Especially famous places, it's about the same. She leaned in, anticipating my next question and preempting it with an answer. "*Then why do mothers go to counseling centers and not hospitals?* Because they think it will remain on their insurance records that their child was sent to a psych hospital and that's a big burden for mothers." In this narrative, the therapist is referring to counseling centers that are private but "non-clinical" and contrasting them to the hospitals that are both public *and* clinical.

Clinical settings offer the promise of standardized quality assurance protocols because they are government regulated and therefore legitimized under health policy and legislation. However, those same clinical settings are also tied to a history of medical institutes and institutionalization, which casts a shadow of stigma over the promises of quality assurance and accreditation. When the clinical setting is also public and governmental, the potential for the negative outweighs the promise of expert care. The stigma associated with clinical care and its mark on medical records when insurance is used doubles such that expertise in the traditional medical sense becomes less valuable. In addition, these counseling centers and non-clinical settings have begun to offer their own form of legitimacy and expertise via certification through private institutes and alternative regulatory apparatuses.

While the gap between the rich and poor will separate clearly given that the wealthy can afford private standardized settings, middle class clients provide a telling sign of the level of stigma associated with clinical services. If cost was held equal, the preference was for non-clinical private settings like counseling centers over public hospitals. This challenges the notion that being on the outside of a system is necessarily debilitating or less preferential. In the case of psychological services like play therapy, the placement of practices both outside the system of health insurance *and* outside the traditionally respected fields of scientific expertise is actually beneficial. These services outside of the system appear more removed from the potential stigma historically linked to the services offered inside of the system.

ARTICULATING VALUE

A few adventurous therapists I encountered chose to open up their own practices. As entrepreneurs they ran into the basic managerial question of establishing costs for services instead of criticizing someone else for paying them too little. Because play therapy was not covered under the national medical insurance system, the prices for services were not fixed. There could thus be great variation in terms of costs for a session of the same length and for a client with a similar diagnosis. This variation often depended on the neighborhood in which the clinic/center was located and the credentials of the therapist.

The variation of costs for private practitioners is not unique to Korea, but it does present a specific dilemma for therapists. Dr. Huh, an articulate and energetic young woman, was one of the few play therapists I interviewed that had chosen to open up her own clinic. She struggled, and still struggles, with how fees can present a barrier to accessing services. She recounted the times parents had responded with, "For 30 minutes, you're asking for that much?!" The main problem she found in managing her own clinic was figuring out how to determine the costs of service so that it would be reasonable both to client and practitioner. After overhead costs are paid, she wanted more to be left over for the freelancing therapists that she hired than what she had earned when she was in their position a few years before. More significantly, she argued that setting prices at a slightly higher level when they originally entered "the market" was important because it "increased value" and "changed the mindset" of clients. Dr. Huh explained that "consciousness in our country is in work. This is work.[3] If you go to the hospital, even if you're alarmed at how expensive, you still go. This kind of consciousness, I think I have to let people know. . .I've been thinking whether we have to be more firm about that." I was fascinated by her articulation of validating her expertise as true work by fixing costs at a competitive level with medical services. To explore further, I said, "I remember when I was thinking about tutoring, I had no idea how to decide on pay in Korea and was talking to my aunts, and I was so apologetic. So for one hour, I'd just say that I'd take however much they could give. And everyone was like, don't do that because. . ." Before I could finish, she added, "It's your price." I wondered if she meant it was my price in the sense of it being my prerogative or whether she meant that the price symbolized my value and ability. She clarified that it was mostly the latter. She then added that this price was also indicative of the amount that I would take responsibility and put time into my work. Dr. Huh added, "When I first began, it was at a social welfare center. . .But I volunteered so if something came up, it's not that I'd miss an appointment, but I'd be more lax. But if I was receiving pay, I'd have to take responsibility and also the client would never miss. If they aren't paying, then they can come or not. But if the parent thinks, 'I'm paying, I have to go'—so for both sides, that's necessary."

Dr. Huh's narrative marks a significant shift in the mindset of therapists from once "just volunteering" in order to gain experience and now reflecting on the management structures of their work and trying to change the very social consciousness that determines who is acknowledged as a worker. It is tempting to think this was a solely profit-driven stance. Though profit was, by her own admission, a concern, it was not the only factor at play. The more I interviewed therapists and conducted participant-observation, the more I found that the scenario articulated by Dr. Huh was indicative of deeper historical roots that contribute to contemporary perceptions of counseling today, and what it means for something to become defined as a form of expertise. Embedded in these questions of reworking "consciousness" is the attempt to gain both social capital and actual economic capital.[4]

Dr. Won, a therapist who has worked in major metropolitan centers like Seoul and Busan as well as far more rural areas of Korea, highlighted this point when she talked about her own experiences in trying to gain employment. She explained:

> In order to get a job, counseling is hard so that's why I left the countryside. Then, I wanted to move elsewhere, and heard they were looking for a psychotherapist so I went [to Busan]. But because my major was in psychoanalysis, using speech to counsel. The first hospital I went to—it was children with autism and I was doing play therapy and psychological intakes, doing things like this. So I had to study on my own about these things that I hadn't learned before. That was my first time counseling children with autism.

I later followed up, asking, "Why do you think there are not many counseling centers in the countryside?" to which she answered with a comparison between rural and urban areas. What struck me was the explanation of counseling being perceived as a "volunteer" or non-professional service. She stated:

> This is just what I've heard. In our culture, we meet and chat without hiding much. Life-long counseling happens in everyday life. So people don't understand why you would pay a professional for that. In the West, you don't really talk about private things, and, if you need someone, you mostly talk about superficial things until you have a closer relationship. They don't really share private things. And in the West, it's more individualistic—this is not a bad thing—so there's a lot of group things and some people could consider that an invasion of privacy. In the West, you take care of your own individual needs and then if you need help, you go to a professional.

This idea was echoed by another therapist later in fieldwork who commented on the double usage of the word sangdam, which can mean counseling when referring to therapy but can also mean consulting in a more general sense.

For example, many parents would talk about receiving sangdam about educational strategies for preparing their children to get into a top college. While there's the pragmatic approach of translating the meaning according to the context of the conversation, the therapist clarified that the word itself used to mean general counseling in terms of any kind of advice. It was not a term linked to occupations or expertise. But with the growth of therapeutic services, people began to think of it as a specialized and professionalized term. Whether in the case of educational consultants or therapists, the professionalization of the term "receiving counsel" has now become an indicator of consulting with an *expert*. It is also important to note the interesting contradiction in Dr. Won's statement above. On the one hand, the notion of residual stigma associated with mental health issues was a pervasive theme during many of the interviews. This would indicate that there is resistance to talking about psychological issues, which contradicts the idea of meeting "without hiding much." In fact, the more prevalent idea in cross-cultural research is that group therapy is more difficult in East Asian communities than Western settings because there is more hesitation to share experiences or emotions with strangers and make their struggles public.[5]

Instead of generalizing Dr. Won's assessment to a comparison between Korean culture and American culture, another micro-narrative of ostensible East/West difference, I suggest that her reflections paint an important and neglected picture of the specific history of counseling in Korea. Dr. Won observes:

> People in the countryside, they say that everyone knows what's going on in all the other homes. So, not really isolated. People are united. In the city, it's more discontinuous—so because we're separated we can do as we please but on the other hand, people don't have much empathy for one another. As things become more Westernized, the need for counseling has developed.

There is an interesting slippage here, for Dr. Won and for many other scholars, between industrialization and Westernization. In the case of contemporary Seoul, she seems to be suggesting that the anomie and discontinuity affects this growing sense of individualism, which empowers people to seek out services to meet their individual needs but also contributes to the sense of anomie that might catalyze or further antagonize any feelings of isolation. The growing need, along with the reduced likelihood of sharing those needs with neighbors, might contribute to the disproportionate growth of psychotherapeutic and counseling services in cosmopolitan centers like Seoul.

Dr. Won also reminded me that people who began to introduce counseling services in the countryside did so as part of a national volunteering program. "I think for counseling to become a career, it took a long time to take root. In the beginning, because they needed counselors, national welfare volunteer programs or other volunteer services. Because that's how counseling first started I think people think counseling equals free. For the memory of that to change, takes time," she said. Another counselor and the head of a community center in a major district in Seoul agreed and added, "A long time ago there was more for a volunteer staff for counseling at community centers, but now there's a shift to licensing and professionalization."

Amidst highly specific and individualized narratives of finding employment and creating a niche in the market of therapeutic services, I could not help but notice the repetitive mention of health care as a system and what it meant for something to be inside or outside of the system. What did it mean for services to be covered, or not as it were, by a universal system? What effects would this have on the practitioners who offered those services? Since many of the psychotherapy programs offered by my interlocutors are not covered by health insurance, I argue that they are all the more a part of the story of health care (as excluded stories often offer insights about the whole picture). Child psychotherapy, and play therapy in particular, is just external enough to the system to posit questions about the benefits and costs to being "covered" and "legitimized" by inclusion in this infrastructure. Rather than foreclosing the possibility for non-clinical treatment to become popular, exclusion has stimulated the emergence of new "marketplaces" and alternative forms of legitimacy.

There are clear advantages and disadvantages to clinical settings (regulated expertise and standardized care, both forms of legitimacy versus stigma). However, this very aversion to public hospitals and forms of stigma *also* poses its own set of advantages and disadvantages. Recall Dr. Ahn, the therapist who I briefly introduced during her discussion of play and work with her mentor. I conducted a joint interview with her and a colleague/friend, a doctor who specializes in physical rehabilitation for children. The conversation went from the comparison between working at welfare centers and being a "welfare-minded" physician to sustaining a working income and explaining how insurance coverage affects accessibility. The physician, Dr. Im, noted that the cost for certain types of therapies is likely to drop and be more accessible to patients if it goes into the insurance pool and becomes regulated. She explains, "In order for treatment to become more popular, people need to feel that it is not only more acceptable to receive that kind of therapy, but that it is a worthwhile investment." When something becomes a worthwhile investment for personal out-of-pocket payments, it is more likely that people will push to have it covered under health insurance.

Entering the umbrella of coverage benefits patients and clients in the sense that costs will be driven down and better regulated within a managed system. Note how quickly logic builds upon itself while also folding in and taking the scaffolding along with it. On the one hand, payment tangibly demonstrates a willingness to invest in a specific service. It lends value to that service. If that service is not yet accepted in "value," it may not be part of a given system (of health insurance coverage, whether it be private or nationally managed). One way of making a case for value and acceptance into such a system would be through increasing service utilization and highlighting people's willingness to pay out-of-pocket for that service. Out-of-pocket payment could thus make a case for coverage and entry into a system. However, there is one major wrench that prevents these cogs of logic from seamlessly flowing into the next. *People would prefer that certain services remain outside of the system.* There is a "trump" card in the deck of values. Social value or the ability to remain free from stigma trumps the value of cost-controlled and service regulated insurance systems. Thus, the extra burden of paying out of one's own pocket is counterbalanced by a greater burden: stigma and fear of "marked" records.

Value is not only constructed and contested by investments made on the client side of therapeutic services. For instance, therapists felt that they ought to be paid more considering the time they spend with each client, whereas doctors are notorious for quick consults. It is easy to take this complaint on the obvious level of salary and crunching numbers to determine relative value. But on a deeper level, the complaint points toward a deeper frustration with knowledge that has been or must be legitimized by a larger regulatory system. On the provider side, the amount one is paid or able to charge indicates the level to which their services are valued by the establishment. This kind of legitimacy is contested and not easily defined. It was highlighted especially during my joint interview with a physician and a therapist. Specifically, the physician was quick to point out that running an establishment required resources other than time and effort on the part of a practitioner.

> **Dr. Ahn (Therapist):** If you think about ENTs (Ear, Nose, Throat specialist/otolaryngologists), they see people for a few minutes so that could be hundreds of patients each day. Compare that with speech therapists or other therapies that take a long time, and then there's a price gap.
>
> **Dr. Im (Physician):** Yes, but you also have to think about equipment costs, purchasing and maintaining equipment. Physical therapy is covered by insurance if the patient is hospitalized. A lot of parents will not invest in speech therapy for their children so it's not competitive yet [with other therapies]. . .It's difficult to follow up and closely inquire. There's the problem of the gap between the *normal* and the *pathological*. For example, if the hospital does not classify the case as *pathological*. For speech therapy, for the therapists, they're not getting paid enough and then for the hospital, it's not worth it because they pay for staff and space and equipment. When you can't use the hospital, you get more services diversifying outside of that setting. Also, licensing becomes an issue...There's

> no national licensing standard or association. It's very difficult to guarantee skills and regulate.

Dr. Im contrasts physical therapy with speech therapy, and highlights how the latter is not valued as much as the former on both the client and provider side. Clients do not feel that speech therapy is a worthwhile enough investment for their children, and thus parents hesitate to pay for such services. Providers have a mixed reaction to this lack of value. For the speech therapists, there is a large degree of frustration for low pay and less respect within the medical field. For hospital administrators, the low pay is justifiable because clients have not shown much interest in investing in this type of therapy and given the amount of overhead costs that go into providing this service, therapists should not be paid that much. Providers in this case can be further subdivided into the actual providers of care (the speech therapists) and the providers of structure (hospital or clinic management that determines how space and time are allocated within the building, and which freelance providers are hired as consultants or full time employees).

In a medical setting, it may even seem cold for a parent or client to weigh whether a service is "worth" an "investment" in such strategic economic terms. But this is precisely the point of interest when studying services and treatments on the periphery. The periphery is not only a useful concept to think about legitimacy in structural and discursive terms, but also a murky area of negotiable value. For example, most parents that my interlocutors encounter would not hesitate to pay for a child's emergency room care or a broken foot. In reality, these services would not be paid for out-of-pocket because they would be covered under insurance but it does not take a great stretch of the imagination to posit that, even if these services were not covered, most of the "clients" would not hesitate to "invest" in treatment. In fact, the very notion of "investment" might not even enter the picture, because the problem and the solution are both deemed *necessary*. It is simply something that must be taken care of, no matter what the cost is. Now, one could approach critique in two ways from this point. The first would be to show how both the necessary and unnecessary are socially constructed and valued according to such constructs.

There is a pragmatic constraint on how people evaluate necessary and unnecessary treatment, much of which is influenced by the degree to which "illness" prevents functional living. But things get much more interesting in the borderlands, where the dividing line between necessary and unnecessary is grey and blurry. For example, where is the line drawn between dental services in a health insurance program that are deemed elective versus those deemed necessary? For example, returning to the physician's comparison between physical and speech therapy in Korea, it is clear that parents do not see speech impediment as necessary and crucial to fix for functional daily life. This is in contrast to the accepted value of physical therapy. Again, from this point I can question why physical therapy is accepted and speech therapy is not. But instead of positioning two categories against each other, I would like to approach this debate from a slightly different angle and look at shades of difference *within* one category. Within speech therapy, what would it take for a problem to become pathological *enough?* Would a lisp be tolerable but not a stutter? Or would both be tolerable enough to wait until "he or she grows out of it on their own or with the help of a tutor"? Contrast articulation or fluency problems with a language disorder where the child has difficulty understanding others or putting words together to express their own thoughts. Would a language disorder be deemed "pathological enough" for out-of-pocket payment to a specialized expert in the feel of speech therapy? These are all questions regarding the process of becoming pathological enough, as my interlocutors alluded to during our conversation.

The power of the public and the politics of epistemological categorization are deeply intertwined in these questions. In *The Normal and the Pathological,* Georges Canguilem illustrated how certain states and traits came to be regarded as normal and others as pathological (1991). Canguilhem demonstrated how these categories came to be constructed in relation to one another rather than taking either as objective fact; the normal and the pathological emerged out of particular social and historical contexts. Michel Foucault, along with contemporary critical psychologists that have offered important ethnographic explorations, built arguments critiquing diseases or behaviors labeled pathological based on the idea that political, economic, and social contexts construct ways of knowing and being.

But what about circumstances where the goal is not to shun the pathological and strive for the normal? What if being categorized as pathological was uncertain? What if being categorized as pathological enough was the difficult task at hand, and proving "enough" pathology had its own stakes? This would mean that pathology was not necessarily the thing to "disprove" against the mainstream norm. Rather, it would mean conceptual frameworks must expand to think beyond what made something pathological. I suggest that a complementary mode of critique would be to ask what the stakes are in becoming acknowledged as pathological enough. In this process of *proving* pathology, what would be the determining characteristic or measure? The doctor in the interview points out how not being pathological enough can exclude patients and practitioners who work in fields that are slightly peripheral to mainstream medical care. It makes certain ailments, behaviors, or types of pain seen as not significant enough for systems to incorporate, managers to address through hiring or salary setting practices, or clients to address when choosing therapy for themselves or their children.

The example used by the physician in the excerpt above contrasted speech therapy to physical therapy but the embedded ideas related to a broader question about the threshold for determining the value of a treatment. Pathology, or the making of the abnormal, can lead to exclusion of populations, but in the context of insurance coverage, this physician who specializes in occupational and rehabilitation therapies argues that her specialty as well as that of the psychotherapist, have been marginalized. Receiving less support transfers the burden of payment to their clients/patients due to the fact that certain ailments are not deemed pathological enough.

Significantly, both interviewees added that this position on the periphery is sustainable if one can open a new marketplace and convince others of its legitimacy. Dr. Im, the physician, argues that practitioners who become frustrated with low pay or lack of respect in medical institutions choose to leave the setting entirely. In this manner, the exclusion of services from legitimized institutions results in "more services diversifying outside of that setting." Practitioners set up shop outside of the "mainstream market" and as popularity increases, the market opens up to include "shops on the periphery." This can result in the eventual inclusion and absorption of these services into the system of health coverage.

In the meantime, services continue to proliferate and find a niche for themself on the periphery of the governmentally regulated medical system. These borderlands are financially viable because clients present a desire and demand for services that are outside of the system's tracking mechanisms. However, while clients are happy to access services outside of stigma-related institutions, they are not willing to sacrifice quality and regulation. Thus practitioners making a living on the periphery are not free from the craving for legitimacy. Instead, they must find or create alternative forms of legitimacy.

ESTABLISHING CREDIBILITY

Legitimacy becomes a key issue here in three registers. Firstly, according to both Dr. Im and Dr. Ahn, the variation in national licensing standards depending on the therapists' clinical background makes it difficult to guarantee skills and regulate practices. Because of limited resources, not all services can be covered under insurance and some are classified as more important than others, either from a financial standpoint or from a quality of life standpoint. Dr. Im points out a key double bind for psychotherapists and their clients. Many of the diagnoses indicate that there is moderate to significant impact on the quality of life for a child dealing with cognitive or emotional disorders, and yet they are functional enough to not require institutional care or psychiatric medication. The cases are "not pathological enough." Furthermore, the services provided by child psychotherapists using play, art, or music are "not clinical enough" to warrant as much fear associated with institutional stigma, but they are also "not pathological enough" to warrant entry into the medical insurance system. Standing on the outskirts of the system benefits therapists because they can dissociate from stigma and operate free from government regulation and price fixing. However, without the legitimacy offered by being part of such an apparatus, these therapists are often dismissed as non-experts. Therefore, they must prove their legitimacy using alternative methods. The exchange between Dr. Im and Dr. Ahn later in the interview highlights this desire to prove their legitimacy, and distinguish themselves from "unregulated" people who lack the quality of training, expertise, and care that they hope to associate with their professions. This desire is more than a matter of prestige; it is the process of differentiation and legitimization from metaphorical squatters on the periphery of a medical system. Thus, even the periphery becomes a contested space of expertise and a place to validate ways of knowing.

Our conversation led to the following exchange between the two practitioners, where they expand on the need for practitioners who are legitimate albeit outside of governmental regulation and those that are illegitimate and unqualified. They identify the problem of a growing niche as the very thing that creates conditions for their success as well as competition from "imposters" who have not put in the time or money to gain credibility from international and local training institutes.

> **Dr. Im:** Competitive play, it's a competitive game. You have to do something other than work at a hospital. So for example, people will open up a center of some sort. Someone might open up a "sports center" where it's like a fitness club or gym. People who graduated from a physical education university become interested in some physical therapy exercises and techniques, so they teach some classes or offer some of those services. But they make sure to not use the word "treatment/therapy." In terms of diversification of services, there's a desire and demand among clients. And hospitals want to meet those needs but they can't, so that's why services go OUT. And then it spreads from that point into different avenues. In America, the boundaries are more defined because of referrals and lawsuits. [Dr. Im had studied or worked in America previously.] There's a combination of issues such as qualifications for therapists and also of surviving in the hospitals. So, physical therapists, for their livelihood, will sell vitamins or provide some other services (like the sports center) so this is how the variety of settings and services increases. Another example for children's physical therapy is a Childcare House. They can ask for Childcare House fees and include physical therapy services as part of the package.

> **Dr. Ahn**: But that's illegal! It's not a real Childcare House. More like a hagwon.
>
> **Dr. Im:** Well, they won't use the name "Childcare House" or at least not the smart ones. Because then that would be illegal and you would get caught. They are expensive, because they can't take hospital insurance.

Though play therapists enjoy their default exclusion from universal coverage because it frees them of institutional memories, they find themselves in a precarious position. They find themselves looking for an institutional surrogate in order to differentiate themselves from completely unregulated entrepreneurs trying to capitalize on the latest child development trend.

Not always included in a system of state licensing regulations or national government databases, play therapists cling to the legitimacy provided by professional associations and other markers of training and certification. Given that these licenses and continuing education credits don't always come from national agencies, and not wanting to be tied to a specific university alma mater should their undergraduate or graduate degree not be elite enough, the play therapists turn to international or "Western" organizations.

Associations and organizations played an important role in validating the work of child psychotherapists. Many of my interlocutors emphasized their certification status through a national association (play therapists in Korea) and/or an international association. They were careful to say how many workshops they had taken, who the workshop leader was, and where they had taken them. Despite the exorbitant costs of international travel, lodging, and conference registration fees—even for middle class Seoul-based professionals—I observed a large number of Korean therapists represented at workshops and conferences in regional and international conferences. I assumed this was simply due to attendees being wealthier practitioners, having family they wanted to visit in those countries, or making a "vacation" out of the business trips. Later, I found out that much of these factors were not descriptive of the women who attended. In examining the policy context, and the importance of finding alternative modes of legitimacy to attach to, the value of attending conferences and workshops and receiving credit from trainers who were known in international networks became evident. Both the international circulation and the Western connections accord Korean therapists with a certain level of organizational legitimacy regarding their knowledge production and occupational practices.

In addition to serving as a mark of legitimacy (whether it be of the mainstream kind found through regulation inside of a system or the alternative kind found on the outskirts), standardization can be thought of as a key construct for functionality. In "Crafting Science: Standardized Packages, Boundary Objects, and 'Translation'," Joan H. Fujimura articulates the key question of "how collective action is managed *across* social worlds to achieve enough agreement at various times to get work done and to produce relatively (and temporarily) stable 'facts'" (1992, 168). In post-Kuhnian studies of science, the argument that facts are socially inflected is not enough. Fujimura's question is significant because the aim is no longer to disprove facticity but rather, to ask how "working facts" are produced. Working facts, like working definitions, are not set in stone but they are important because they must be cooperatively agreed upon and stabilized for enough time for groups to get work done. Fujimura argues that a key conceptual component in dealing with "collective work across divergent social worlds *and* fact stabilization" is the standardized package (169). A standardized package is the combination of theory and technology, adopted by members of multiple fields for the purpose of building new working definitions in research. Like D.W. Winnicott's concept of "good-enough," a standardized package allows for work to be done when complete consensus on facts is difficult. Standardization as a conceptual tool for establishing legitimacy and standardized packages is both temporary and flawed. But it is meaningful and useful because it creates a space for productivity. Fujimura's explication of "standardized packages" in studying science as concept development and practice is most relevant in rethinking knowledge production in a classic academic, laboratory, or research setting. But when thinking about the work of knowledge production among my own interlocutors, I must also ask how standardization resonates with stakes in both knowing *and* being. Play therapists must standardize their concepts, practices, and protocols for a long enough period of time to stabilize their work and expertise. In doing so, they also have more at stake than producing knowledge and getting work done; they become *workers*—they come into being as legitimate experts who are producers and practitioners of knowledge. Thus, standardization becomes a method and concept for stabilizing identity and the work linked to it, both of which are contested and not taken for granted when living on the periphery.

Being on the periphery of a system can actually be a positive factor for clients who feel more comfortable going to therapy at a less institutionally associated place or believe that paying out-of-pocket and avoiding insurance coverage keeps sessions off the record. On the provider side, this ambiguous peripheral position calls for therapists to establish "legitimacy" in other ways: by working for a doctor at a physician-owned center, opening their own business if they feel confident about their credentials, or being attentive to membership in local associations or transnational networks. Many of the therapists told me about their training and certification experiences, and the research that supports the efficacy of their treatment during our interviews, performing an iteration of legitimization as they spoke to a Korean American researcher.

While shadowing many of these therapists during workshops and conferences, I served as both interpreter and photographer, running around taking snapshots of the therapists with their American trainers, including some of the heads of major training institutes. Some of the other international therapists chuckled in amusement and others in annoyance, as each Korean therapist had to take a separate photograph in addition to the standard group photos. I did not think much of it, as most tourists visiting another country might be prone to frantic photo-taking. But months later, as the issue of legitimacy unfurled in the themes of the interviews, I began to realize how important it was for them to post these pictures along with their certificates on the walls of their clinics or on their websites. These were the seals of standardization that signified an alternative legitimacy to governmental inclusion and regulation.

The play therapists I interviewed distinguished themselves from illegitimate practitioners in these new marketplaces by stressing the quality of their training. Their attendance at workshops, photos with certificates in hand, and ability to convey their expertise to potential clients is crucial to survival in this emerging "niche market" of mental health—of treatment centers and clinics that cultivate "psychological well-being" or therapists that use play and the arts to treat social, emotional, and psychological problems among children. When dealing with transnational networks of experts, it is not enough to say that knowledge or knowledge producers circulate. This is certainly the case as therapists travel to and participate in international conferences and training workshops or share their knowledge through written email exchanges or videos of sessions.

But so much more happens. On a local level, circulation, standardization, and re-standardization are always occurring. In the excerpts from government officials and local practitioners that I have highlighted in this chapter, the legitimacy of new knowledge forms come to the forefront of a complex system of stakes and investments. These stakes and investments weave in and around the already present and stable lattice of governmental structures or health policies. But when they are denied access to these stable structures, workers (and their work) are not stopped. Rather, productivity branches out—it goes out and diversifies.

Work (and workers) live—and make a living—in the borderlands.

Chapter Four

Achieving Intuition

If legitimacy can appear in many forms, then the marker for quality is no longer limited to the realm of government regulation. Left to govern themselves (and in some respects, happy to do so), play therapists tap into alternative modes of governance. These alternative forms of governance hold equal or greater sway because they tap into the legitimizing power of cosmopolitan striving—and global belonging. Korean play therapists attend training workshops alongside practitioners who come from North America, South America, Europe, Africa, Australia, and Asia. Through these encounters and through shared experiences in acquiring new knowledge and skills, the Korean therapists embed themselves in an international network of trained experts. Thus, governance and legitimacy via professional associations simultaneously offers a sense of broader global belonging and more opportunities for mentorship by trainers in a field that does not yet have regulatory bodies in local or national government.

Professional branding through global belonging sets trained therapists apart from untrained entrepreneurs while also underscoring their new role in society as experts at the intersection of child development and mental health. This notion of expertise is one that weaves together a complicated web of anxieties and desires. Individual narratives of expertise are interwoven into national narratives and vice versa. Concepts such as "globalization" or "neoliberalism" take on robust meaning when concretely anchored in the specific case study of Korea and the stakes of real people—of women who struggle to establish their professional place in a new work sector, and of workers who struggle to cultivate their expertise on the local, domestic, and global stage.

This chapter examines expert-making processes that require individual management of intuition-cultivation as well as organizational management of program fidelity across sites around the world. Though specific in nature, as all case studies are, the reflections in this chapter offer practical and concrete articulations of anxiety and desire in ways that complement theoretical critiques of socio-cultural phenomena. In the fine grain detail of everyday worries and problem solving, and in the voices of a small group of female play therapists, I hear echoes of broader debates that have captivated scholars and pundits. It is my hope that the analysis of specific and concrete narratives will show the incredible work (and play) that goes into knowledge-making and expert-legitimizing.

CULTIVATION

In a small but tidy room at a community welfare center on the western end of Seoul, Dr. Ahn was preparing to meet with her client. I had been asking her about her expectations for the session. I wanted to understand what ran through the mind of a therapist before a session and how she prepared herself for what, by design, seemed unpredictable. We chatted briefly but before I knew it, it was time for her client to arrive and for me to leave the therapy room. Because of the structure of the center, students (therapists in training or researchers like me) could observe through a one way mirror that ran alongside the wall. I made myself comfortable in the adjacent observation room. This room could sometimes be shared with the parent of the child receiving therapy, so that a grandmother, mother or father could observe and ask questions during a one on one consult with the therapist that followed each session. Today, the child's mother had decided to wait outside in the lobby rather than in the observation room so I was alone with just my thoughts, a pen, and a notebook.

I opened my Velveteen Rabbit-like pad of paper, flipping past the neatly organized and meticulous notes of the first few weeks of fieldwork to the more recent pages filled with sporadic, scribbled ideas and observations. A clean page finally appeared and I clicked my ballpoint pen several times before putting its point on paper. I started scribbling a few basic notes about the setting for the session and the activities that would be included.

I looked through the mirror at the wisps of white clouds painted on sky blue walls. It was an inexpensive but important touch that added an element of warmth in what was essentially an empty room with a few rectangular cushions to sit on. In fact, the clouds and painted walls were the only thing that distinguished this room from most other settings in which this particular type of play therapy was conducted. This was one of the key selling points of this particular style of therapy because it was easier to address fidelity to the model when settings remained consistent, whether families were being seen in this welfare center across the parking lot of a government subsidized apartment complex or in a posh private clinic. It also underscored that the power of therapy was not in the size or resources of a center, but rather, in the quality of the interaction between therapist and child. Program fidelity was not about dosages, instruments, or settings but about the quality of the therapist and their ability to interact with the unique needs of every child and family. Program fidelity depended on expertise embodied in the heart/mind of a trained therapist.

I could see Dr. Ahn beginning the session with introductory games and songs. Her client, a distracted and slightly agitated youngster seemed much improved from the original sessions, when all 30 minutes would be spent trying to bite or hit the therapist. My aim was not to evaluate the effectiveness of this therapy, as that was something my interlocutors themselves were in the middle of doing as they practiced clinically and collected data for their own research projects. Instead of evaluating efficacy from the lens of a supervising therapist, I paid careful attention to the hybridization of work and play, and how both therapist and child negotiated these hybrid forms of work/play. Embedded in this question of work/play was the collision between things that had been dubbed "natural" or intuitive knowledge such as playful interaction and things that required training (for the therapist) or treatment (for the child).

What female play therapists did (work with children, playing and counseling) had everything to do with who they were (women in contemporary Seoul, experts on the periphery). As I observed sessions and interviewed therapists, I listened to their personal and professional reflections. I felt a rhythmic pendulum like swinging between articulations of experience and intuition. It occurred to me that the pendulum might not be swinging from one pole to another but rather, circling around a hybrid form of experience and intuition—a kind of carefully cultivated intuition.

Intuition by its very nature is supposed to be innate. One might imagine a salesman demonstrating how "intuitive" their user interface is to a potential customer. The implication in this sales pitch is that the customer need not worry about the strain and stress of learning because using the product will come naturally. And yet, for play therapists, intuition is a vexed term. The therapists study theories and strategies, read text after text, and receive supervision after supervision to refine their techniques. They create session plans and reflect on ways to improve after clients have returned home. But planning only goes so far in the world of play (and in the world of therapy). Therapists are constantly thinking about ways to adapt and revise their session activities based on what the client needs during the session. In short, there is a constant feedback loop of thinking, trying, working—of cultivating. For the therapist that can go through the feedback loop quicker and quicker, the session becomes more seamless and less awkward; he or she seems to be adapting to suddenly presented "wrinkles" in the session plan so quickly, "it seems natural." In short, the therapist works so hard at cultivating their expertise that he or she eventually achieves intuition. The catch then becomes the articulation of this hard earned intuition in a world where parents, peers, and policy makers may use words such "seamlessness" and "natural" as justification for little or no pay. Cultivated intuition or intuitive expertise is both coveted and feared ground for it serves as the mark of a seasoned professional as well as the ways in which their professional status may be subsumed under assumptions about natural mothering skills (particularly since play therapists are predominantly female in Seoul) or good natured volunteering via child care. It becomes all the more important, then, to articulate the intense *work* of play and how deeply *cultivated* such intuitive expertise truly is. Cultivated intuition is the result of legitimized knowledge infused into or laid on top of sensibility, adding intentionality to instinct.

For therapists who work/play, thinking and feeling happen at the speed of interaction. What does it mean for thinking and feeling to occur within every interaction and at such a rapid speed that one does not have time to parse out which is which? During my interviews with Dr. Ahn, the theme of expertise as a "feel for things" became especially prominent. A truly experienced therapist was someone who knew so much that they developed an excellent "feel for things" and depended less on rote memorization or rigid protocols. This idea of cultivated intuition and developing a "feel for things" was indicative of both the content and method of this study. It formed a large part of the therapists' core narrative about finding a place in the child development and mental health sectors while also exposing an important aspect of field methods. "A feel for things" was an important and often repeated phrase among the therapists I interviewed. It also resonated with me personally as I grappled with reflections about anthropological field methods.

While preparing to go into the field (wherever that may be and however "field" may be defined), cultural anthropologists often find themselves writing proposals and creating timelines. These are exercises that serve multiple functions, from acquiring funds to outlining major research questions. And yet, every anthropologist knows that such plans are flexible and if anything, a researcher who is more committed to the basic tenets of anthropology will be ready for change and adapt to life as it happens in the field. "Thinking as you go" among play therapists paralleled anthropological anxieties about the need to plow forward with both adherence and adjustments to "the plan." At stake for both the therapist and the anthropologist was a need to be flexible, while also finding ways to articulate how flexibility was the mark of a *more* seasoned expert rather than a free-styling lay person. Just as play therapists find themselves needing to articulate all the work that goes into play, so do cultural anthropologists often find the need to explain participant-observation as more than "hanging out" to those less familiar with the discipline.

Evelyn Fox Keller discusses this idea of "a feel for things" and its connections to gendered knowledge production in her biographical work on scientist Barbara McClintock, *A Feel for the Organism* (1983). The play therapists I worked with were using "a feel for things" as a term that indicated something so completely anchored in preparation and yet, so resistant to rigid planning. During one interview, Dr. Ahn explained how a session might be planned with certain activities and dimensions of attachment in mind, but might be suddenly altered when the client entered the room. She paused and said, "Of course, you have to watch the flow, watch how the activities are flowing." She made me remember one particular session at a community center where I had been helping her as a volunteer for group play therapy. Because this was at a community center, the families and children were "non-clinical" cases and receiving an introduction to play therapy. Some of the children would later be identified as cases needing referrals for individual therapy, but at the time, this group was the perfect example of why play therapy presented a de-stigmatizing alternative to other kinds of therapy. Play therapy could enhance parent-child relationships even for children who had no clinical diagnosis. Additionally, in more intense settings and with more intentional session plans, play therapy could be a viable treatment for children who had been clinically diagnosed.

Dr. Ahn asked me to recall one specific morning at that community center. A few families called the morning of a group session and said they could not make it that week. This changed the number of participants and the kinds of group activities that could be done since they had been specifically adapted to work in large group settings. The therapists met 30 minutes prior to the start of the session and discussed how they could still offer the benefits of specific activities that aimed to facilitate parent-child attachment, while adapting to the new (smaller) group size. Dr. Ahn then reminded me about another day, a day when it began snowing so the community center was colder than usual. The other volunteers and I took out flannel blankets and placed them on the floor so that the families could have a warm place to sit upon entering. As they transitioned from sitting on the floor to an exercise that was meant for the families to move around the room to interact more dynamically, the therapist integrated the blankets into an activity where the parents pulled the children around on makeshift sleighs. It allowed the therapists and families to transition more smoothly between activities and eliminated the need for clients to wait for the volunteers to clear the room of the blankets. It also allowed focus to remain on interaction rather than on setting up or cleaning up.

Dr. Ahn remarked, "So sometimes that's how you can make changes. Just because you plan or prepare ahead of time doesn't mean you have to stick to it. You think, oh it'd be good to do this activity. And then, oh this activity might be better. If you think that, you change it." Dr. Ahn's sentiments were echoed by Dr. Kim who explained to me that there are days when "you've gone in prepared but then there are situations where none of the activities seem to be working. Then, I have to think of the activities I know and quickly adjust trying one by one. Because we're not robots." Dr. Kim described trying to make sense of the sudden flurry of thoughts such as, "What should I do? Why isn't he or she doing it?" that swirl in her mind as a child presents unanticipated reactions to an activity. She reflected:

> It's not about doing everything and it's okay if you throw out one of the activities or instead you can replace with another activity and that works. I think that's *more* correct. In the beginning, it was just about following the schedule because I stayed up until dawn planning it, but it's not that. You have to follow the child, so you take the activities but adjust to the child. And if that activity seems like it's boring the child, like we've done it a few times and the child has grown tired of it, then quickly you transition to another activity. Like if you planned this activity for three minutes or five minutes, and you think we *have* to do more or longer for a few more minutes. That's how I *used* to think, but now I can adjust more and there's more flexibility.

Like so many other therapists, Dr. Kim, Dr. Cho, and Dr. Ahn highlight their growth as professionals and experts by the ability to become *more flexible*. In doing so, they frame their work as highly cultivated through years of practice involving rigorous planning and learning when and how to abandon those plans. Expertise for these workers is measured by greater variance and the ability to adjust. And the more rigorous planning and learning one has invested time in, the more one should be able to demonstrate flexibility.

I recalled scenarios I had observed during individual sessions. For example, when a child became overexcited and dysregulated from the excitement of a certain activity, the therapist would rethink the next activity. For some children, an engaging activity where the therapist would blow soap bubbles and ask the child to pop the bubbles as they floated through the air would quickly evolve from giddy excitement to overwhelmed stimulation—or as therapists often referred to it, dysregulation. If the child could regulate their level of engagement, the activity would be simply delightful and allow for transition to an equally stimulating activity. But many children were sent to play therapists precisely because they had a difficult time engaging with others during playtime; they would either withdraw in a way that made a simple game of "Hot Potato" come to a standstill or get overexcited in a way that made it impossible for both child and co-players to *enjoy*.

For those reflecting critically on psychology, this may seem like just another manifestation of the constant pressure to self-discipline and regulate but I want to emphasize that this was not just a matter of children feeling like they had to be perfectly amiable or compliant. For readers unfamiliar with play therapy and more familiar with critical theory (descriptive of myself prior to embarking on this study), it might be tempting to analyze the therapists' narratives and session notes as simply constructing the abnormal and creating yet another arena for self-discipline (not to mention profiting off of the creation of new categories of pathology). But as I worked alongside families and therapists during my time in the field, it became clear—at times explicitly so and at times more of an intuitive gut feeling—that these children's struggles were not simply manifestations of socially constructed categories or arenas of discipline. A therapist's ability to assess the child's level of regulation was crucial to his or her expertise and capacity to meet the child where they were while also helping them to learn how to regulate their mental, emotional, and physiological reactions. If the next activity had originally been planned as another high-energy activity, the therapist would revise on the spot by slowing things down and using a more subdued activity that would require more focus. The new activity could be a game like "peanut butter and jelly"—a "Simon Says" of sorts, where the therapist says "peanut butter" in a funny voice and the child responds with "jelly" in the same tone or voice as the leader/therapist. To an outside observer, blowing bubbles and repeating words with silly voices might seem equally delightful ways to establish connection and enjoy play but if thought about more deeply, they require different skills. "Peanut butter and jelly" requires focus and matching, asking the child to wait and listen carefully to the tone of voice that their partner uses in order to replicate. It requires a greater level of concentration.

Dr. Ahn reflected on what goes through the mind of the therapist in just a matter of seconds as a therapist veers seemingly off course by choosing a different activity than the one originally planned. As a seasoned practitioner and supervisor for newer therapists, Dr. Ahn notes how much cultivated intuition plays a role in differentiating the master from the apprentice. She explains:

> You're thinking as you do it . . . That's why experience is important . . . other therapists that I'm working with, for example in this group program, well there's a wide range in terms of levels of experience. How many sessions they have had led impacts how smoothly, how instinctively, how naturally they do it. And so there's a big difference. Even if we all decide together to do the same activities, I see out of the corner of my eye that a group is not going very smoothly. And that's the difference that experience makes.

The same game played last week without a hitch could incite anger or anxiety in a child this week. She explained to me that this could be due to something as simple and mundane as a child coming to therapy after a toy broke, or after a bad day at school.

When underlying issues surface during a session, sometimes triggered by an activity and sometimes seemingly out of nowhere, the therapist must quickly adapt. Adapting and responding "almost intuitively" is what becomes the marker of high quality play therapy and high quality (that is, trained and experienced) play therapists. This cultivated intuition is one that comes from session after session of experience; it is this experience that allows a therapist to attune to a client's needs and respond in a flexible manner. And yet, flexibility is only one side of the expert coin. While honing one's skills, therapists must also maintain fidelity to training models and modalities. As much as therapists underscore how a seasoned therapist exhibits a kind of intuitive flow, they are equally if not more careful to emphasize how much training goes into this level of responsiveness.

Dr. Huh, a therapist who had been working for nearly a decade, reflected on her own transformative journey from skeptic to believer. She said, "In the beginning I didn't think it was much of anything and was not sure if it was really even therapy. It looked so easy and I thought, who couldn't do this? But after doing it, it is a really difficult and strenuous thing." In her reflections, as well as those of Dr. Ahn and many other therapists that I interviewed, the expert was the one who learned "the program" the best. "The program" was often a specific model or style of therapy that required a series of workshops, trainings, supervisions, and credits. The best learner understood the elements of "the program" well enough to replicate across settings while retaining fidelity to the model. And yet, the best learner was also the one who refrained from painting "the program" into a corner. This expert could achieve and enact the fine balance between flexibility and fidelity.

COMMUNITIES OF PRACTICE

Many of my interlocutors who had established themselves as experts within their own communities of practice, spoke of the fine balance between achieving intuition and articulating more than "just intuition" to outsiders. One strategy of articulating expertise to new and potentially skeptical audiences involved the mining of established fields of expertise. For example, play therapists in Korea would weave in theoretical constructs and findings from neuroscience and developmental psychology along with clinical social work. Therapists had to not only demonstrate their expertise but also craft narratives that explained how a true expert who seems to "just play" was actually the one who had worked the hardest. The appearance of natural, intuitive work could only be achieved through careful and intentional cultivation. This was a mantra repeatedly uttered to one another, to semi-insider/semi-outsiders like me, and to critical outsiders.

Dr. Lee, a therapist in her late 20s and one of my youngest informants, recalled a conversation with a colleague who was working at a play therapy program held in a local church that provided programs for families in the neighborhood. During the course of the program, her friend kept telling her about various misconceptions people had about therapists' activities because "it just seemed so leisurely" compared to "serious therapy." Dr. Lee echoed the sentiments of many of the other play therapists I interviewed, saying, "I think there are misperceptions and false understandings like that, where people think we're just playing. And that's why on the one hand, [it seems like] anyone can do it easily. But once you do it, it's actually difficult." As they address these misconceptions with parents before and after each session, the therapists gain experience (and expertise) in *articulating* therapy in addition to *doing* therapy.

"To explain is actually a tricky thing. To what extent do I need to explain? Do I need to give an academic explanation, like what I'm learning in a graduate program? Plus, there's not a lot of time so it can be burdensome. But then, if you don't explain, it can appear to just be play, and a bunch of activities. I still worry about this question," said Dr. Lee. Her colleague, Dr. Shin, raised the same issue when she said, "My supervisor told me *not* to answer all the questions, to just set the limits of relevance to that particular session. Partly because it's better to provide more structure, and also because it sets more of a tone of expertise instead of the kind of random conversation you have with a neighbor." What is most striking here is that the therapists strive to strike a balance between providing enough information to explain that this is not just play while setting the boundaries of their consultations to prevent it from becoming unstructured like a conversation one might have with a friend. It is not only the quality of information dispensed by the professional therapist that defines his or her expertise, but also the quantity that structures the relationship between the giver and taker of therapy.

Because the play therapy community was small—growing, but small—practitioners relied on their social and professional networks heavily to find practicum sites, job opportunities, and to follow up with prospective clients. With programs replicating and practitioners encouraging peers to begin the certification process, a great deal of energy was focused on implementation and execution. And yet what struck me as highly reflective for a "start-up" group just beginning to get a handle for its emergent practices was the therapists' constant conversations about articulating their expertise adequately and capturing data. The first was an issue of communication and the second fell in the research and evaluation category; both were subcategories under one general anxiety: the need to legitimize a new form of knowing and doing. It was not simply about legitimizing a finalized version of practice, though. Even though therapists were seeking out ways to legitimize themselves and their practices, they were still growing, learning, and revising.

The process of becoming an expert through involvement in networks and institutions is often described in limited terms that rely on a hierarchical linear narrative. In reality, the development of expertise that I witnessed among the therapists was much more blurred between professional and personal relationships, where the group of practicing play therapists in Seoul was so small that they often relied on one another for career development.

Along the way, some became friends and supervisors and senior practitioners became mentors to therapists in training. And the path to expertise was also a more spiral-like trajectory rather than linear. They constantly reflected on ways to do and say therapy better. They reflected on their own, with one another, and with me.

Jean Lave and Etienne Wenger have argued against the notion that learning occurs and exists only within the mind. Instead, they contextualize learning as a practice that is just as much about "participation in the social world" as it is about acquiring specific forms of knowledge (1991:43). Learning can be thought of as a process that occurs within a community of practice, rather than an independent endeavor that only makes use of others in order to facilitate an internal change in the mind. Lave and Wegner argue that all learning is part of a community and situated in culture. Furthermore, the community is not only one in which the ratio of old timers and newcomers changes, but also one where the community of practice itself changes (115). For example, a group of therapists becomes a community of apprentice therapists, certified therapists, supervisors, and trainers while the therapy itself and the definition of that community also morphs. People become the community and the community becomes a reflection of the people.

Lave explains that "apprenticeship training may equally well be characterized as an inductive method of learning, which would lead to the acquisition of general cognitive skills, although skill acquisition might have different sequence and rate characteristics than skill acquisition in school" (1977, 177-178). Here, Lave is emphasizing the notion of apprenticeship in response to much of the earlier scholarship that assumed apprenticeship in trades such as tailoring does not facilitate the transfer of cognitive skills (for example, in understanding mathematic concepts in measurements for tailoring) the way that formal schooling would because it was more "concrete and task-oriented." Although the style of learning is inductive and not as explicit as a math class might be, Lave argues that learning by doing is an alternative to the more acceptable notions of learning and then doing. She also states that apprenticeship organizes learning activities in informal but still structured ways, suggesting that structure is not exclusively available in formal education (1982, 182). Lave and Wenger further develop this notion of apprenticeship as a crucial way of learning and establishing communities of practice in less institutionally bound contexts. Lave and Wenger's concept of "legitimate peripheral participation" (1991) is a concept that aptly describes how therapists become a part of the community of practitioners in Korea and part of broader networks dispersed throughout the world. It also provides a perspective of participation and collaboration that recognizes the different scales of integration and responsibility, while identifying them all as legitimate members of the community.

There are degrees of learning while doing in this case, where the therapists gain expertise partly through formal education and partly through apprenticeship. This combination of formal and informal learning opportunities is nothing new but what is striking about the case of play therapists in Korea is the transnational nature of their apprenticeships. Because initial cohorts of practitioners were dependent on established training institutes, associations or organizations outside of the country, apprentice and master were often located oceans apart. Many of the therapists I shadowed were trained at workshops during overseas travel. They would return home, and in the early years before there were digital copies and compressed zip files, therapists would ask clients for permission to record videotapes. These tapes would be packed carefully in manila envelopes or cardboard boxes and sent to organizational offices abroad. Trainers there would review the clips and then send notes back to practitioners eager to strengthen their skill set. Supervision took place transnationally and through the very literal circulation of ideas by way of moving people (therapists traveling to workshops across the pond) or moving things (videotapes).

Although this was logistically and sometimes financially difficult to manage, it was worthwhile because it afforded the therapists a protocol for certification and created an alternative mode of governance and regulation. Therapists might have had professors, supervisors, or mentors who gave them regular feedback and who were locally available but because certain styles of play therapy were so new during my time of fieldwork, I found that many therapists were reliant on professionals who were located abroad.

Toward the end of my fieldwork, local expertise had grown to the point that supervision and training could be provided within the country. Since then, communities of practice have grown dramatically to the point that practitioners are no longer dependent on the feedback of outsiders. However, what remains relevant for this part of the workforce is the complex relationship between dependence/independence and local/global participation that developed during the early years of these therapeutic programs. Reliance on trainers based in the West provided an option for supervision that met a practical need while also presenting the extra credit (nay, credibility) of belonging to a necessarily transnational network. Furthermore, the visits to international conferences and training workshops gave them a chance to learn alongside practitioners from around the world. In the absence of local governance, practitioners of an emerging therapeutic modality were able to find legitimization, standardization, apprenticeship, and global connectedness.

Throughout the international conferences I participated in and observed during my fieldwork, I noted how the global network of certified practitioners and apprentices was growing. The practitioners who came from various continents shared their experiences, and specific speakers were brought in as special guests. However, growth meant more than the rising number of participants in the network of practice. The practice had grown to the point where it began to expand beyond its own network. In fact, the speakers' presence and the substance of their talks signified the need for the program to be explained and justified to outsiders by using research, theoretical frameworks, and other scholastic pools that often constitute a stronger foundation for evidence-based practices.

GLOBAL CONNECTEDNESS

After one of the international conferences had concluded, I stayed behind to serve as a translator for a group of therapists who had come from Korea to take an advanced-level workshop. I heard and saw the daily struggles my interlocutors went through, and what emerged as a recurring theme was the basic need for the therapists to be acknowledged as experts or trained professionals in order to be a useful service that someone would pay money for. This identification as expert would provide therapists the means to earn enough to not only contribute to their daily expenditures but also allow them to travel and remain active in international networks. Thus, cosmopolitan striving and global belonging offered an alternative mode of legitimization. But this was only a temporary solution. After all, they had to live and work in their home country and no amount of belonging in an external network would replace acceptance and acknowledgment from a local public. Domestic belonging and governance would eventually be necessary in order for the programs to take root. Taking root in Korea would create long term viability of practice, and providing funding for practitioners to continue to travel and connect with their peers from around the world.

The great irony of this example of transnational apprenticeship and global network-building is that it stems from local context. It is local context that pushes practitioners to seek resources outside of governmental regulation. As with any emerging practice, early adopters often find ways to be mentored or affirmed from more established experts in other locales with more established histories. But the very same local context that pushes Korean play therapists out toward global networks is also the context that creates, validates, and encourages such longing for global connectedness.

In 2010, Sook Jong Lee and Kevin Hewison penned an introduction to a special issue of the *Journal of Contemporary Asia*. They begin "Introduction: South Korea and the Antinomies of Neo-Liberal Globalisation" with the following:

> It may seem altogether too late for a special issue on globalisation and South Korea. After all, many well-known economists and not a few government spokespersons have praised South Korea (hereafter Korea) as one of the

> world's most successful examples of late capitalist development and rapid adaptation to the trajectory of globalisation. Indeed, with relatively poor natural resources, various Korean governments have long pursued an expert-led industrialization strategy and Korean conglomerates (*chaebol*) have become global companies and are at the leading edge of technological innovation in electronics, automobiles, shipbuilding and so on (181).

By now, it is true that globalization conversations seem almost passé because they have been around for administration after administration and through multiple economic cycles. Korea's export of electronic goods and other "expert-led industrialization" products has long tied together domestic political economy with global networks. Aside from trade networks crystallized through the distribution of electronics, automobiles, and shipbuilding, citizens also tout the notion of "Korea for the world; the world for Korea" in discussions about Hallyu or the Korean Wave. Hallyu began in the late 1990s and the term itself was coined from Chinese characters that literally translate to "flow of Korea"; the phenomenon describes the popularity of Korean music, dramas, and films in other parts of the world (initially in parts of Asia). With these flows of Korea disseminating out to the rest of the world, came the opening up of a new market for exporting images and sounds.

Globalization in this context, whether in the export of things or ideas, sets the world stage to receive Korea—Korea for the world. The local for the global. But simultaneously, globalization means that the world is valued as it takes root in Korea—the world for Korea. The global for the local. One obvious example of the intermingling of global and local value-making is the dominance of English tutors and tutoring centers in Seoul, where most students learn English from an early age. As Park and Abelmann have argued, mothers who are savvy in navigating public and private educational resources readily display their "cosmopolitan striving in a global order" (Park and Abelmann 2004). Such mothers (and their children) are perceived as more than good citizens in the local context; they are cosmopolitan beings in a global order. These displays of cosmopolitan and global citizenship, as well as basic displays of localized class status, are reproduced in education settings as well as in therapeutic settings.

Associations for play therapists were growing during my time in Korea but for the majority of my research study and particularly in its early years, nearly all therapists touted their connection to some form of international group; their membership and certification from such groups leveraged these connections as well as the regulations stipulated by these groups to earn certification to become regulated and trained experts in the eyes of their peers and clients. The individual narratives I analyzed during my research serve as articulations of expertise, staking claims to knowledge when their roles as experts are not a given. It is also the reason why their international networks of training become so important to stress as part of the experience one needs to become an expert.

At one of the most popular private clinics the play therapists worked, I noticed how the website featured blond haired blue eyed children smiling, and a subpage explaining the center owner's ties to training institutes in Europe. Meanwhile, all of the families I saw milling around in the lobby had black hair and brown eyes. Traversing to another part of town, I would hear therapists talking about their latest experience at an international conference where they had received training credits or presented results from their local study to an international audience. Bookshelves of volumes written by doctoral students and professors working in the subfield of play therapy were easy for me to read because they were in English. Some were placed next to translated versions and others stood alone. At times, it made sense given the therapist's proficiency in English but at times, it seemed odd to purchase long tomes in a second language that would be barely read given the strain it would take in comparison to reading similar material in Korean.

In the world of emergent expertise, this striving to be part of a global order was not simply the abandonment of local status for a greater global identity. It was the display of cosmopolitanism as a creative solution to the lack of ability to display locally regulated expertise. In connecting to the broader global order through basic concrete things like collecting books in English, displaying certificates from international institutes, completing apprenticeships under the supervision of a US-based practitioner, or traveling outside of the country to Europe, Korean play therapists were able to create an ad hoc legitimacy in the face of a lack of locally-based regulating structures while also tapping into a broader context of deep local appreciation for participation in global flows.

Bridging the micro and the macro, the play therapists I observed grappled with all kinds of ways to achieve expertise. On the one hand, they managed their own reflections to understand how thinking and feeling was part of their careful cultivation of expertise. They then crafted those reflections into narratives that articulated just enough—not too much, not too little—to convince clients or critics of the work that went into play therapy. They explained their seemingly seamless "flow" within sessions as the kind of flow that could only be demonstrated by truly skillful laborers. It articulated labor and expertise for therapists who were not wholly accepted by society as such while also encouraging parents who felt lost and hopeless.

Interactions and "homework" for parents and children might feel frustrating, marked by the staccato rhythm of disrupted flow stemming from the inability to play that had first brought the children into therapy. But with a little persistence, parents and children could labor together to eventually achieve flow. Through work, and with the support of therapists who were also attempting to find flow in their work, parents and children could return to the thing that was never the departing place: a natural ability to bond through the delightfully spontaneous openings provided by play.

Chapter Five

A Good-Enough Proposal

Everyone I met was working hard to play. The therapists thought about how they could do and "talk" play therapy better. They thought about how they could hone their skills to present a kind of seamless facilitation, and also about how they could explain their profession to others. If they could run a session that constantly anticipated the needs of the child, they could eventually create a space for the child to experience the spontaneous joy found in play—and in so doing, experience that joyful moment of work. Parents also worked hard to play. They worked to support therapy sessions at home and to learn the concepts and techniques. They worked to build healthy bonds with their children, and made time to work alongside their children as they sought to discover the joy of play.

The parties involved in a play therapy session did not fall neatly into mutually exclusive categories of Therapist and Parent. The roles were blurred for several reasons. First, the short-term nature of many of the programs I observed required the mother to become a lay expert. As sessions progressed, a therapist would teach the caregiver the same activities and concepts she had been using to treat the child. Of course, the skills taught to the parent would be accompanied by a more brief and simplified version of all the theory and research that the therapist had been required to learn during graduate school or certification. Still, the transfer of expertise from therapist to client lent itself to more open-ended power/knowledge dynamics. It also complicated the critique that the therapist simply leverages expertise as a means to securing continuous profit streams.

Although the term "clients" included mothers, fathers, grandparents, and other caretakers, I refer to "mothers" often in this chapter and throughout this book because they comprised an overwhelming majority of the clients I observed. Furthermore, the role of mothers was of particular interest for the therapists because, as women, they felt they needed to articulate a clear difference between their professional role and the role of the mothers.

This is a core difference between how my interlocutors see their subject position as a therapist (who just so happens to be female) and the subject position of a mother bringing in a child for play therapy sessions. While expertise seemed to be circulating and transferring hands constantly, a distinction was made between learning enough to support play at home in between treatment sessions and learning enough to become a certified professional who could charge fees for their services. Parents needed to be informed by theory enough to support practice but the emphasis was on application. Meanwhile, therapists needed to be adept at both theory and practice, and convey that skill to the wider public.

Another key difference between therapists and mothers is the time and resources therapists put into developing their skills throughout their careers. Staying on the cutting edge of the field helps to define them as dedicated professionals, rather than lay people. Part of this dedication to professional development is a desire to engage in reflection and receive constructive feedback. Therapists arrive at training workshops with the intention of becoming better professionals so a certain level of critique is not only acceptable but actually desirable. Critique is part of the feedback mechanism that allows professionals to advance in skill level. To some extent, openness to critique also exists when a mother makes the careful and conscientious decision to bring their child to therapy and consult with a therapist. However, mothers arrive as willing collaborators intent to learn as much as possible in a short period of time, but limit their engagement for that short period of time. Still others were described as "just wanting the therapist to fix their child so they can go home and get along with their child better."

Dr. Kim explains how there are some mothers who "take it really well, but like children, all mothers are really different." She continues:

> So for some mothers, when you make an observation, they're like, "Okay I think I really am doing that and acting like that to my child, but I won't do that anymore." And mothers that cry because of small things they did—they see how it really influenced the child and they're so sorry so they start to cry. But then other mothers, it goes in one ear and out the other. And once, they go outside [the center or clinic] it's the end. So for those children, the duration is really long and I mean, they improve, but it's different from what would have happened if they had done some of it at home. Like the child will really like it, but the mother doesn't want to do it so then it returns to the way it was. So things like that, depending on what the mother does, there's variation. But still, it's better than not coming at all. It's much better than a mother who doesn't come at all, but depending on what you do after you come, there's also quite a difference.

When therapists make observations, they do so as professionals consulting with clients and not as peers providing advice. Many therapists emphasize that their intention is never to assume the role of a mother but rather, to stand in between the space of mother and child in order to help facilitate their interactions. Here, it is not a matter of the therapist teaching the client how to be a mother since the therapist may not be a mother herself and even if she were, has no desire to tell another women how to parent. The client has already come in as a mother and the therapist does not purport to have that expertise. Instead, the knowledge and skill transfer has to do with the specifics of the program and type of therapy, rather than exchanging roles. The boundaries between the roles are blurry but there are subtle and important differences.

WOMEN'S WORK

Alongside the differences which revolve around dedicated time and energy to learning and articulating the connections between theory and practice lie the similarities between the roles of mothers and therapists. Many of these similarities have to do with overlaps that occur due to the gender of the therapists.

Initially, the issue of gender was not a major focus of this study. It was not that it was any less important than a myriad of other themes that appear within anthropological discussions. But given the scope of the project, I did not explicitly set out to discuss gender in my interviews. In part, I was following the lead of the therapists who identified more with their alma mater or level of experience than with their gender. And yet, the more we spoke and the more we explored, I noticed how the play therapists' professional narratives often became entangled in their personal reflections about family. This was due to many factors including the fact that they were a part of a growing workforce that was dominated by women. There were also constant slippages between professional and personal stories that toggled back and forth between reflections as a therapist and reflections as a working mom. These kinds of slippages were worth noting because the therapists were in a position where they felt pressured to be both Good Therapist and Good Mother.

As they grappled with ways to best articulate that they were Good, they found a way to be good-enough and to articulate good-enough as an alternative to the conversation about good vs. bad or normal vs. pathological. Faced with gaps in resources and oftentimes not quite sure how to balance efforts, these women found solace in creating working-solutions—solutions that could be created in good-enough spaces that were not perfect nor meant to stay that way forever but were functional enough to create spaces for creative problem-solving.

All of the play therapists I spoke with during my time in Seoul were women, many of whom were middle class and also mothers. Their stories about work incorporated their reflections about parenting, even though most of my questions and prompts were questions about the state of the child mental health workforce in Korea. Yet when I noticed that they were going back and forth between lessons learned in trainings and at home as mothers, I began to ask follow up questions. I noted how my interlocutors were especially careful to underscore the *difference* between their personal and professional roles, but ultimately ended up articulating their growth and development in terms that relied upon *hybrid* narratives that thought out the role of therapists and mothers in more complicated and entangled terms.

I recall one particularly poignant conversation with Dr. Cho, whom I met for coffee at a small café near a university in Seoul. She explained, "People who've only briefly studied [it] think you just have to follow the program but in actuality you can't do it like that. And that's why the therapist's role is important." "When it looks really easy is when the therapist is doing a good job and making it seem natural. And because it's smooth, it looks more like a mother-child. It looks easy. But you know, it's really difficult," continued Dr. Cho. It was a brief statement, but because the usually soft spoken Dr. Cho stressed her words, I paid careful attention. In that simple statement, she affirmed what other therapists had noted. There was no perfect adherence to a protocol because the better the therapist and the more experienced the practitioner, the less she would be dependent on a protocol and understand the meaning of interaction more deeply. She would be free to go with the flow. She would adjust so quickly and deviate necessarily from plans that she would make it smooth and natural-looking. Such adjustments required the ability to deviate from plans. If done deftly enough, the trained therapist would appear to be so in tune with the child that it would appear natural—as if a *mother and child* were "just playing" together. Making it seem natural made it look more like a mother and child in comparison to the highly work-driven interaction between a therapist and a child.

Dr. Cho added, "It looks easy. But you know, it's really difficult." She knew that this is what people thought of play therapists, and challenged this notion with her counter-narrative of labor. Thus, she was articulating the *work* of play for child therapists. But the point of reference was the "mother-child" who would be playing naturally rather than the "mother-child" who had come to her as clients. She slipped into this reliance on an idealized and naturalized understanding of play between mother and child even as she herself tried to produce a counter-narrative that went against naturalized expertise for female therapists. Her clients were actually mothers and children who could not make play seem natural. They struggled to enjoy the delightful and spontaneous exchanges many take for granted in a childhood filled with "Patty-cake" or "This Little Piggy" or any other local equivalents.

In her classic essay, "Is Female to Male as Nature Is to Culture?" Sherry B. Ortner argues that the pan-cultural or universal subjugation of women is often situated in discourses of biological or genetic determinism (1972, 9). Women become associated (and closer to) Nature as men become markers of Culture. Ortner goes on to argue that the divide is often nuanced. In this case, women are not solely "to Nature" and men "to Culture" but rather, women become relegated to specific parts of culture. Culture in the private sphere becomes associated with the domain of the domestic such that women are given the socio-cultural role of childrearing and holding the family together. The responsibilities of managing the private sphere are acknowledged as important socially, but less so than the opportunities available in the public sphere. Culture in the public sphere becomes a domain associated with males and masculinity, creating an imbalance in socio-cultural responsibility and participation.[1]

Anthropologist Sharon Traweek adds that the identity of knowledge producers impacts the relationship between what individuals produce and how they produce it (1999). She writes, "Affect and gender are significant components in the division of labor in laboratory research, as well as in decision-making, dispute-making, and leadership styles that are part of the whole realm of power and tradition in scientific research" (540). Gendered roles are infused in the narratives of knowledge production, for all its moments of success and failure. For play therapists in Korea, this argument is also relevant because they are mostly women who are not always taken seriously as legitimate experts.

Like many of her colleagues, Dr. Cho had spoken at length with me about the difference between professional and personal roles to ensure that articulations about being a therapist were not mistaken for articulations about being a mother. And yet, also like many of her peers, her reflections could not be kept apart for too long. It was in this back and forth that I could see the therapists still working out how they might embrace both roles in their life and give credence to their hybrid forms.

The therapists I worked with noted that you could never teach someone who hated children to care but that did not mean all who loved and cared for children would make adept therapists. The qualified therapist was not defined by being a perfect practitioner or a perfect mother. In fact, therapists were clear to mention that there were many wonderful therapists who, for various reasons, were not mothers nor intended to be in the near future. Instead, a professional was someone who could take good instincts and cultivate them so that they could be experts. Their knowledge resisted categorization as wholly innate or wholly learned, but rather, lived in the in-between space of cultivated expertise.

Gendered articulations of cultivated expertise became crucial as my conversations with the therapists evolved. They pointed out several key ways in which gender entered the picture. First, if the therapist was not a mother herself, she had to position her expertise on grounds other than firsthand experience. Second, even if she were a mother, who was she to be able to help someone else? This was not a parenting class nor was it the kind of "general chatter" two mothers might engage in as they chatted over coffee while sharing stories about their families. In fact, therapists' discussions often turned into defending one's expertise in order to move away from a naturalized interpretation of play therapy. The stress on how much work was done, how hard work was, and how long it took to do good work became all the more important as elements to producing a stronger counter-narrative to naturalized knowledge and expertise.

Dr. Lee, a young therapist around my age, joked with me, "I study children and am a therapist so I think I have a responsibility to do a good job later raising my children. Like if something goes wrong, uh oh!" I laughed at first, but it made me wonder about the intersection where the pressures of being a good-enough therapist and of being a good-enough mother collided. Not yet a mother, Dr. Lee focused on how her growth as a therapist had influenced social relations in general, particularly with other members of her family. She explains:

> You can't help but think about it. My undergraduate major was child development and as I went into that [in my graduate studies], well not just that but also child psychology—the first assignment is to think about our own childhood. I had homework like that and even if you didn't want to reflect on the past, if you looked back, you start to think about it a lot. When I was a child. Especially because [play therapy] is related to attachment, I think about the kind of attachment I formed with my mom. And actually, what was so good was that, personally, I don't like to reflect too deeply, but as you do [therapy] you have to really look deep inside so I got to do that as I did my homework and learned a lot. Things I didn't know about by doing that. . .And so, things like that. Also, my relationship with my mother and father have improved. That I put more effort to be more conscious and aware. Our family is not the type where we chat a lot, not that we have bad relationships at all, but we're just like that. But now, I talk to my mother a lot more and I make an effort to talk to my father a lot too, just things that aren't a big deal but to just chat. And with my younger sibling, I'll ask her to go to the movies with me. In junior high and high school, there was nothing like that. So I started to see that and think about it more.

Therapists like Dr. Lee were careful to separate the play they do at work and the play they do at home in their narratives of therapy, but their experiences with understanding and exploring the dynamics of attachment in social relationships continued to cross those seemingly strict boundary lines. It seemed that the expertise of the therapist could easily transfer into generalized and ostensibly universal concepts about child development, and thus carry over into one's personal life. But they were hesitant to state the converse lest it dilute their claims to legitimacy and specialized expertise.

The idea of professional wisdom flowing into personal growth is not an uncommon idea as many professionals begin to incorporate what they learn through work in broader observations and experiences outside of the office. What complicates this idea is the guilt brought on by leaving the child to work with "other people's kids." However, the reverse was not necessarily true; while having positive personal experiences (raised by a mother who played with you a lot, or having already raised one's own children) *might* be somewhat helpful, it could never replace the strength of proper training if one was to become a quality therapist. Thus, the chief source of ambivalence came from going *out* to work/play rather than bringing work/play *into* the home with them. In these narratives, the therapists articulated their identities as women in the home and women in the workplace.

BRINGING WORK HOME

Play therapists remain keenly aware and extremely intentional about separating the professional and personal value of play therapy. Describing play in the context of training professionals means that specific theories and practices are transferred between master and apprentice; expertise is honed, crafted, and cultivated.

Toward the end of a treatment, when the child makes enough progress, parents are often asked to join the sessions and work alongside the therapists. During the last few sessions, play therapy skills are transferred from therapist to parent so that they can continue their progress at home. The goal, therefore, is never to keep a child in therapy for the long term or to create dependence on an infinite number of sessions. (It needs to be stressed that the therapists understand that these short term programs are not something that would be proposed to treat severe cases that required pharmacologic treatment or long term counseling. Given the growth of cases that were falling somewhere in the "middle ground" of Korean medical services in structure and in cultural acceptance, there was a need for a type of therapy that could address a variety of other issues contributing to the child's inability to enjoy social interaction. In this niche, play therapy and play therapists set up camp.)

From my outsider perspective and more patient/client advocate-inclined subject position, this short-term structure was so appealing. From my quasi-insider perspective, I wondered how this would work for therapists trying to build a narrative around expertise in a specialized workforce. Wouldn't the transfer of skills from therapist to parent essentially be the equivalent of the therapist working themselves out of a job? This might seem like a nonsensical question for others in the mental health field, particularly those that work in any kind of outpatient setting but the reason this seemed so crucial for this particular group of therapists was because of the stakes they had in defining and establishing a *new* set of practices. Since so many still did not recognize what they did as a profession, the transfer of skills to parents (ie, lay people who had no previous training in these fields) could further confuse the public in understanding what special set of knowledge or training the therapists had—and what special set of services they could provide to the public. It was in this context that I began to realize how crucial the differences in articulating play at work and play at home was for the therapists. Conversations between trainers and apprentice therapists differed from those between therapists and clients, largely due to the differences in purpose. Even though both pairs represent relationships where one side is attempting to facilitate the transfer of skills[2] to the other, the trainer's goal is to cultivate a professional whereas the therapist simply aims to provide tools for parents to use in their everyday interactions with their children.

Perhaps it was because of this constant transfer of skills between therapists and between therapist and client that the public often slipped into the private for my interlocutors. In my interviews, I often noted slippages between professional and personal reflections, weaving in and out of the spheres of the therapists' own lives. For example, recall Dr. Ahn, one of the therapists I had observed and interviewed earlier in my months of fieldwork. At the time we spoke, she had two children who were "almost all grown up." She had also advanced to a stage in her career where she was consulting with parents as well as teaching, coaching and mentoring. As we sipped tea during a casual interview, I began to share some of my own reflections on going to various workshops in the US and how I felt awkward because I lacked both professional and personal experience with young children. She responded:

> If you've raised a child, it's probably helpful but there's a different problem. Just because you've raised a child, it doesn't mean you're mature [as a therapist]. For me, it was the opposite. I was thinking back [to raising my own children]—Oh I should have done it like this. So just because you've raised a child some time ago doesn't mean you do it all well. So if I was single, unmarried and never had a child, it doesn't mean you can't do it. You're getting experience. So in general if the person is warm and soft, if I was brought up that way and received that kind of childrearing, then those kinds of people can actually have an easier time. Not about whether you have or don't have a child. But rather, if I possess those traits. Also, as you keep working, you change and learn how to do it.

There were many oscillations between expertise as mother and as therapist, and between expertise as inherent and cultivated. For example, Dr. Ahn stated that certain personal experiences like raising a child helped when working with children. But she then placed a much higher degree of emphasis on the professional experiences of therapists who kept working and clarified that being a mother and therapist were two different things. She talked about the possession of traits as integral to a person's character but also emphasized that people can change, learn, and grow. When she remarked, "Just because you've raised a child some time ago doesn't mean you do it all well," she was once again reminding me that experience as a mother does not equal experience as a therapist. In telling me this, she was saying that women who are not mothers should not be judged as inferior therapists while also emphasizing once again that there is a level of professional investment one must make to be a trained therapist.

Dr. Ahn's articulation resonated deeply with conversations I had much earlier during preliminary fieldwork. I recalled one specific moment when I had been sharing reflections with a licensed therapist at a workshop in the US. I told her that she would probably be so much better at a particular workshop activity given that she was both a therapist and a mother—and I was neither. Pausing momentarily, the young woman then responded, "Actually, as a new mother, it's kind of weird to suddenly be playing with someone else's baby." For her, it was an adjustment to play the same games she played with her daughter with other people's children.

A few days after my conversation with that therapist, one of the trainers leading our workshop series commented that she herself had no children and that that was not the therapist's role. My own assumptions about skills coming easier to those who could draw from their personal lives and experiences were slowly being challenged and would continue to develop into a complex tension between the therapists' own roles and identities in professional and personal spheres. Therapists' expertise would become articulated in terms far more technical, and yet, still be embedded in ideas of possessing warm and nurturing traits. Thus the narratives and counter-narratives they produced were never wholly purified versions of "nature" or "culture" but always a *blend* of instinct and learned behavior. Being situated in the domain of the psychological allowed such hybrid narratives to make sense, as developmental psychology in this context was always-already situated at the interstices of the biological and the social.

When therapists in Seoul talked about who takes care of their own children while they were at work, they raised similar issues. Dr. Kim was about to go on maternity leave at the time of our meeting. We had begun to discuss the general trends in caretakers who brought children to therapy or who participated in family sessions. In the past, this group would be composed entirely of mothers but in the past few years, more fathers, aunts, or grandparents had become involved. This was partly due to the fact that more women were working. Dr. Kim said, "If you just look at us, our baby, and it's not like I come out to work every day but I do work, so his grandmother (father's mother) watches him. There's a group of seven to eight children his age in the neighborhood and only my son gets watched by his grandmother; the rest of the children are take care of by the working *ahjummas*." She made several differentiations in contemporary childrearing scenarios, all resulting from women like herself working more. The children were lucky, like her son, if they could be watched and reared by a relative like their grandmother—implying that this was because the grandmother would be more invested in how the child grew up than a non-family member. Others would be watched by the *ahjumma*, who was often at home as a housekeeper primarily and babysitter by proxy. She continued to speak at length about the impact of mothers working and what that meant in terms of the woman experiencing mixed feelings of pride and guilt from being at work rather than at home with her child.

A slightly more guilt-ridden narrative came across during my interview with Dr. Yoon, also a working mother and therapist. She was one of the most articulate interviewees I had spoken to at the time, who often incorporated academic concepts and theoretical frameworks in her explanations. She was not necessarily a formal person, and we had already had several exchanges prior to this interview so I knew her to be a friendly woman, but the format of this meeting as an "interview" brought out more professional "speak" from her. Part of it may also have been due to the fact that she, along with many of my interlocutors, had seen me at their workshops and conferences and this, coupled with my introduction to them as a graduate student, made me viable as a colleague. I tried to de-formalize the interviews and switch to a conversational style, as many were nervous that it would be a journalistic experience where they had to answer as representatives of their field of expertise. I mentioned that I had the chance to hear a presentation given by a well-known American therapist's daughter who told the audience about how she had grown up playing some of the games with her mother as she was developing therapeutic programs.

Dr. Yoon's eyes lit up and she shared several stories about her own family. Dr. Yoon nodded in response to my random ad hoc comments and said that she, too, had "tested" out some activities at home with her own child. Dr. Yoon explained that when she did these activities at home, her young son became interested in her work. "I'm sorry to my child because I go to work and [when I come home] my child says, 'Mom, did you play with other kids?'" she said. Dr. Yoon continued, "So doing this therapy has also affected me personally in child rearing. . .For my child, I want to do well. Like if I get angry, now I have insight and think about why I was like that. So next time I won't do that." Becoming a therapist did not suddenly make her want to "do well" by her son as that was already a desire beforehand, but it did seem like her professional experiences had caused her to reflect more deeply and more often on the dynamics of her own mother-child relationship.

Working as a therapist made her more committed to paying close attention to her child's development and fostering healthy bonding. But working as a therapist was precisely what was keeping her away from her child. She did not want to give her best at work to other children and somehow fail to carry over new insights and skills into her role as a mother.

I had so many conversations like this where therapists tried hard to articulate their role as professionals in a new workforce that was supporting parents and children in Korea. They attempted to articulate how play therapy could support healthy relationships between parents and children and ultimately, support the healthy social, emotional, and psychological development of children in Korea. As they wove together narratives about their training and experience, they began to integrate their own personal experiences as parents and as children. It was in these moments when I saw how the therapists were struggling to be good-enough both at home and at work.

The reason that being good-enough was a meaningful struggle was because effort was important. Effort symbolized work and work still needed to be done. Joy still needed to be found and the kind of joy in child's play (whether their own child or the children of others) could only be achieved through work. Achieving Good in its perfect terms as the Good Therapist or the Good Mother was impossible but it was dangerous to not try at all given all that was at stake. A good-enough model for supporting parents and play therapists needed to be developed.

GOOD-ENOUGH

Therapists, parents, and children were working hard to find a way to play. Prior to this research, I had always taken play for granted as something that came naturally—as something that provided sweet relief from work. But as I studied the work of play therapists, I became more attuned to just how hard it was to play. I thought back to my first observations in the field when I noticed the beads of sweat accumulating on a therapist's forehead during the course of a single therapy session. In the following months and years, I began to see all the complex issues that contributed to the therapists' desire to be acknowledged as workers. I saw how important networks were for practitioners in an emerging field.

In establishing their communities of practice in Korea and beyond, a group of women had begun to piece together resources and connections to build a viable network for circulating tangible and intangible assets. In my time working alongside these women, I found myself encouraged by their resourcefulness and resiliency. The same seemed true for parents, for children, and for the various people I encountered as I traced the growth of play therapy in Korea.

The therapists were well aware of criticisms about their work because they themselves had the same criticisms—although, in their minds, the criticisms stemmed from "faux professionals" that were contributing to the perception that play therapy could be implemented without training, certification, or regulation. I admitted that I had entered Korea with pockets full of all kinds of citations from the literature about the social construction of pathologies. But as I have alluded to several times already in this ethnography, I saw so many families feeling relieved to find a therapy that might work for their children. To say that a child who could not talk to peers, who could not interact with his or her own parents, and ultimately, who could not enjoy play was just an example of constructed pathology seemed unfair. To say that all of the therapists were driven by sheer desire for profit also seemed unfair. Upon closer inspection of their working conditions and salaries, it also seemed just plain inadequate as an analytical approach.

Play therapists simultaneously acknowledged something was wrong but did not add to the stigma around pathologies in mental health. In fact, because their treatment was play-based, it became the type of thing that would "do no harm" for any child that participated in sessions offered in nonclinical spaces such as community centers where parent-child programs were regularly offered. At the same time, the therapists were constantly reconfiguring their narratives and practices in order to differentiate between play therapy activities used in nonclinical family programs and play therapy activities used in the context of a therapeutic session.

The people involved were neither pathological nor normal, and neither good nor bad. They were all trying to move forward—to grow as professionals in therapeutic expertise or to grow into healthy parent-child relationships—while accepting that there would be no sudden moment when the Good light bulb would flash on. It was in this context that I began asking what it meant for therapists and parents to work toward something knowing that was not a perfect solution but rather, an important *operational* one. Like the "working definition", the "good-enough" understanding of being a professional or being a parent allowed them to work towards a better healthier way of being without being paralyzed by the sudden demand of perfection. The point of parents and children enrolling in therapy was not to churn out the forever Good Mother or the Good Child. And the point of training and regulation was not to churn out the forever Good Therapist. Everyone involved would still be prone to error, as all humans are. And yet, embracing the "good-enough" would allow them to move forward rather than letting the dichotomy of Good and Bad rule their lives.

As therapists reflected on this notion of operationalizing their work through the "good-enough" they began to reflect on its meaning in their professional *and* personal lives. What would it mean for one's mental health to be good-enough? For a mother to be supporting her child's development in a good-enough way? And for a therapist to guide a wide range of families to receive good-enough support? If perfection in this lived reality is impossible, and good is often dismissed as a monolithic category derived from subjective perspectives, then what are we left with? Do we leave it all behind as an attempt to defend the unique individual against all social norms? This is where the concept of "good-enough" gained traction.

Typically, "good-enough" implies a kind of subpar standard where everyone acknowledges its lackluster sheen but accepts it as a kind of last resort. But the concept of "good-enough" in play therapy refers to the term as described by D.W. Winnicott, a trained pediatrician and therapist, who later became an acclaimed object-relations therapist in Great Britain. Winnicott provided a form of psychoanalysis and an approach to treating patients without inferring that everyone must comply with a specific social norm to be deemed mentally healthy. In fact, he once wrote:

> It will be noted that I have not used the word "normal." This word is too well tied up with facile thinking. But I do believe that there is such a thing as psychiatric health, and this means that I feel justified in studying society (as others have done) in terms of its being the statement in collective terms of individual growth towards personal fulfillment (190).

Among his many theoretical contributions, Winnicott advocated creativity (which works well in advocating play therapy and efforts to foster play as part of healthy child development) and acknowledged the inherent imperfections of each of the participating individuals that constitute a relationship (Winnicott 1971). For Winnicott, it was not about the Good Child created by the Good Mother or the Good Therapist. In fact, he coined the phrase, "good-enough mothering," as the best that one could hope for—to create a "good-enough" situation to prevent any major inability to grow and relate to others (Winnicott 1971). In short, he encouraged people to create safe and nurturing spaces that did not stifle growth, but at no point did he encourage delusions of perfection.

This concept of the "good-enough" ability of imperfect beings is striking when thought about in the context of my interlocutors' words. According to Winnicott, a good-enough mother would provide for the physical and psychological/emotional needs of her child as those needs shifted throughout the phases of child development. This awareness could be conscious or unconscious, and was significant in defining the mother-child relationship more flexibly. Rather than the mother determining the precise direction of the child's growth, the parent would change and attune to the developing needs of the child. The mother could then be viewed as the person creating a place and space for the infant's projections, thus providing the child with the ability to adjust to life as a more independent being.

The good-enough mother is different from the perfect mother or the Good Mother, because she "starts off with an almost complete adaptation to her infant's needs, and as time proceeds she adapts less and less completely, gradually, according to the infant's growing ability to deal with her failure" (14). Her "failure" here is not the kind of failure one thinks about when thinking of an absent or distant parent but simply the "failure" of the parent to do everything and be everything to a child who has grown from dependence to independence. In order for independence and resiliency to develop, the parent must embrace the kind of productivity that emerges in the wake of "failure" and the kind of hopefulness found in being good-enough.

The failure to respond to everything or to provide everything is inevitable, but it is this limitation that allows the infant to grow and develop in a world where he or she will have to deal with failure in the world at large. The mother unconsciously fails in a gradual way so that there is no sudden shock in dealing with shortcomings. The therapist unconsciously fails in a gradual way where they learn that seamless flow is achieved only when plans are challenged during the course of a session.

Good-enough is no longer the failure to reach Good. Friction is no longer the foe of Flow.

Chapter Six

Disruptive Translation

The child therapists in Korea leveraged flexible notions of fidelity as they adapted knowledge and practice. Adaptation began to take place as all members of a community of practice adjusted to the one another's feedback. Flow became bidirectional as local practitioners reported to trainers their own findings; those applying theory and converting concepts into practice described areas where manuals and frameworks did not seem to translate well. As word spread about different styles of play therapy, flow became even more multidirectional. Therapists across the globe began to implement theories and practices, share experiences and ask questions. They discussed constant refinement of skills with one another through written correspondence, casual conversation, and more formally at conferences.

Like my interlocutors, I traveled back and forth across multiple sites during the course of the study. As I moved between the cities, regions, and countries, I generated a flow and friction of my own by virtue of my own constant displacement. I realized that therapy programs circulating from "West" to "East" were actually traveling and making meaning through mutual exchange. There were cases where the flow was more unidirectional but in those instances, meaning often felt one dimensional. In cases where flow was bidirectional or multidirectional, program adaptation took on more nuanced meaning. Circulation of concepts and practices depended upon local relevance and local feedback as much as it did the guidance of originators and regulators. Translation as a mediational event between parties came to represent a more powerful way of facilitating flow and viewing friction as part of the meaning-making process.

I came to understand how transnational knowledge production went beyond oversimplified understandings of taking established products and simply adding window dressing to make it palatable to local consumers. I came to see how every successful therapy plan included reflections about the kinds of knowing, thinking, feeling, and doing that happen between parent and child, client and therapist, trainer and apprentice, and between micro networks within international macro networks.

TRANSNATIONAL KNOWLEDGE-BUILDING

New practitioners and their trainers understood that practices had to constantly adapt in order for a standardized program to stay alive and have impact every time it landed in a new locale. Adapting to diverse norms about play, parenting, and pathology was critical to maintaining the flow of this model across sites, ensuring its relevance as a "universally" applicable way of helping children and families. At the same time, the legitimacy of programs and of the therapists' tie to standardized evidence-based therapies hinged upon the network's mutual commitment to practicing the same kind of therapy and resisting pressures to change practices to the point they became unidentifiable. In short, the therapists grappled with the need to change the program enough to be locally relevant while upholding universally identifiable characteristics of the model.

Science studies scholar, Michel Callon, has long challenged the linear chain of innovation in innovation theory, which often describes the process as a series of events: research → invention → development → innovation → diffusion (Callon 2007:312). He differentiates between formulas that *predict* and approaches that can be revised to *accurately describe*. Oftentimes, in a unidirectional paradigm of program adaptation and translation, everything is aimed to not only predict but also to only be successful if predictable. That is to say, standardization requires a degree of predictability. While results vary and every client is unique, a standardized program should conform to a degree of predictability if it aligns with the implementation formula. But if we think about translation and adaptation outside of a predictive (and prescriptive) paradigm, we might consider a more accurately descriptive form of translation. If translators resist predicting meaning through a word for word equivalent-finding algorithm, they can look at broader contexts and ideas as they appear in action. The objective of this kind of translation is to arrive at something that accurately reflects the intent of the speaker but also describes content in always-new ways. Keeping content always-new ensures that meaning stays alive.

In tracing the transnational program adaptation of play therapy and the cultivation of roots in Korean society, I began to see how much my task was to look at how the formula for training therapists was being revised to more accurately describe (and treat) conditions rather than seeing the formula as predictive of how much could be relaxed for local relevance (that is, how much could be "compromised") without losing fidelity. Translation is the process by which an object changes during movement; these changes do not necessarily imply a compromise of authenticity (Latour 1999). Fidelity to meaning or to accurate description should not be mistaken for fidelity to predictive formula. In fact, through the circulation and movement of objects and meanings, references take on a life of their own—a process of transubstantiation where the sign "appears in place of the thing" (64). Bruno Latour writes, "We never detect the rupture between things and signs, and we never face the imposition of arbitrary and discrete signs on shapeless and continuous matter. We see only an unbroken series of well-nested elements, each of which plays the role of sign for the previous one and of thing for the succeeding one" (56). This concept of fluid movement and continuous shaping and reshaping of knowledge was reflected in the ways in which therapists circulated information and experiences.

In some ways, every iteration of the therapy's program included a series of unbroken elements that constantly substituted new for old. And yet, it would not be accurate to say that what I observed was devoid of rupture. In fact, I found the flows of knowledge and practice in this study to not only contain ruptures but to also integrate productive "breaks" in order to facilitate circulation. Instead of seeing ruptures as barriers that halted the process of circulation, interlocutors used them to pause and reflect more deeply on core meaning and their collaborative translation of that "more accurate description" of play and of therapy.

The psychotherapeutic exchange is one where the client is presented with the challenge to put their feelings into words, articulating emotion and thought. Ruptures between the pure intensity of thought or feeling and the articulation of that experience into speech already calls for a kind of translation where there is no pre-identified equivalent. And so there are pauses, and pauses can signify ruptures where one concedes nonequivalence but finds deeper meaning and more accurate description. Ruptures appear as barriers at first but if they can be viewed from a more hopeful and productive place, they can also be opportunities to experience freedom and creativity. Extend the need for translation from thought/feeling to speech within the individual to the need for mediation between therapist and client as they attempt to understand one another. Then multiply again the iterative layers of translation and the possibilities for rupture when examining large-scale transnational adaptations of psychotherapeutic programs.

Viewing rupture as a potentially productive moment rather than as a sigh-worthy barrier allows practitioners to interpret the process of translation as a continuous seamless process. Difference across sites becomes less problematic and more emblematic. This is because the adaptation process of a psychotherapeutic program that begins in one part of the world and lands in another *necessarily* involves both repetition and difference.[1] Repetition invokes adherence to a method that has been proven effective. A great deal of work goes into making the case for a program's efficacy, enough to merit movement and circulation. Thus repetition is a necessary part of passing along a program that individuals believe in. The program must *necessarily* change in order for meaning to be preserved and for the program to continue to exist. It must be tailored to each community in order to be relevant, so relevance and fidelity must come together in the proper scaling up of a training model.

In the play therapy programs I observed, repetition included circulation through several countries and continents. Critical elements like the classification of the components of play into relationship-building factors remained the same across contexts, including the management of standards and references to cohesive conceptual frameworks for understanding socio-emotional development in children. At the same time, changes *had* to occur in order for the program to make sense and be effective in a new environment. A new activity could come about as the practicing therapist thought of variations to activities they had learned in workshops and refashioned according to what made sense in their own community. But "new" was actually quite relative because a therapist who really understood the underlying concepts behind the playful activities demonstrated in a workshop could identify those elements of structure or nurture in longstanding playful activities common to Korean culture. For example, for many generations, it was common for Korean grandmothers and mothers to carry their children on their backs. So the functional "piggyback" ride was quickly adapted into a quieter activity that focuses on aspects of a nurture-based dimension. While carried on the back, mothers could look side to side to catch a glimpse of their child's face, creating a subtle version of "Peek-A-Boo." The therapist would show the mother how to turn her head, first to the left and then to the right. In doing so, the mother would "surprise" the young child on her back with a word similar to "peek-a-boo!" The activity would become a hybrid of concepts and traditions, new to both the lead trainers and the home institution. From one perspective US trainers could be seen as adapting to local Korean customs and from another perspective the original Peek a Boo activity was adapted to a more functional version for its "new" local context. Thus, an old game could then be introduced as a new activity within an international network of therapists.

Adjustments were clearly being made all the time, but that did not preclude the expression of many therapists' anxieties. A primary concern in discussion of how a program will be adapted and implemented is this notion of "violating fidelity" to the original program (Kumpfer et al. 2008). Questions about how much change is permissible without violating fidelity range from worries about superficial changes such as aesthetic presentation to more profound anxieties around structural shifts (Castro et al. 2004, Resnikow et al. 2000). While there is no complete agreement, the general consensus seems to be that change poses the threat of compromising the original program. It is only a question of how much loss can be risked or tolerated in order to achieve cultural appropriateness.

As I continued to work alongside my interlocutors, I reflected on many of the observations made by the play therapists. I began to look at program adaptation and translation itself as modes of co-producing knowledge as it circulates, rather than risks to violating fidelity. And, if this co-production could be seen as necessarily involving all stakeholders, it would be behoove program adapters to "recognize and involve all stakeholders in the translation process" (Nuyens and Lansang 2006, Sussman et al. 2008).

Translating the program across cultures includes more than merely putting the concepts into Korean words or finding equivalent activities. Concepts are held constant through repetition across sites, cities, and countries. But in this case, repetition cannot merely be wrapped in different flavor coatings of difference. Instead, repetition and difference must fuse together to produce something that demonstrates adherence to the "original" program and something that is wholly appropriate to the new context. As anthropologist Timothy Choy describes, "Translation, in its conventional sense, allows knowledge to be communicated from one person to another even though they speak different languages. If, however, we assess translation not simply as a communicative act but, rather, as a mediational speech event, we glean another insight" (Choy 2005, 10).[2] Bringing this mediational (rather than communicative) definition into the exploration of transnational program adaptation reminds us of a desire to accurately describe rather than simply prescribe. And this large scale mediational understanding of translating therapy also mirrors the kind of mediational event that is depicted par excellence in the act of play. Play as a kind of mediational speech is produced in interactive spaces where the rules of the game "rupture" to allow room for the kind of spontaneous joy that forms and strengthens the bonds of relating to one another.[3]

LOCALIZING RELEVANCE

If transnational knowledge production is about the co-creation of knowledge through mediational translations between practitioners, then local relevance is the same side of the coin as global applicability. I turn now to descriptive notes I recorded during the course of fieldwork, beginning with chronologically earlier notes from a session in the US and following with observations from a session in Korea just months later. Pay close attention to what might be organized in the bucket of "similarity" and what might be labeled with "difference" as you read the two session descriptions.

Session A:

A small girl with wavy brown hair, pulled back by a colorful plastic hair band adorned with flowers, enters the empty room slowly. Her small steps are tentative, but her eyes dart around the room with telltale curiosity. She quickly glances around, looking for a few tiny hints that might tell her what today's games will be. Still holding her therapist's hand, she takes a quick glance back over her shoulder to check that her mother is still standing in the hallway. Mom smiles, gesturing reassuringly with a small wave of her hand. This is not the first session so the girl does not seem scared. She recognizes the fun lady she played with last week. But she still seems unsure about why she is here or what she is supposed to do. She looks up at the lady for any indicator of what her afternoon will be like. Her therapist is a friendly middle-aged woman with blonde hair pulled back into a neat ponytail, dressed comfortably in business casual khakis and a loose button down shirt. She smiles but turns her attention to walking toward the center of the room with her client. They sit down and begin. The therapist notes all the healthy beautiful attributes of the girl, from the ten wiggly toes and fingers to the tiny freckles on her cheeks and the wavy curls that swoosh up at the very end of her tendrils. Over the next 30 minutes, they move on to other activities, ranging from a hand-clapping activity like Patty-cake to a cotton ball race (blowing a cotton ball across the room) and a makeshift basketball game using balled up newspapers. They wind down with a snack, as the therapist feeds her five-year old client miniature pretzels and orange juice. Together, they lean in to listen to the sound of the crunching noises, and enjoy the last few moments of the session. Finally, they sing a song and close the session, holding hands and walking to the door. They open it and find Mom sitting on a chair in the hallway reading a magazine. They reunite briefly and while another therapist watches the little girl, drawing pictures or just chatting, the therapist and mother enter the room. Because the mother was watching through a video feed in another room (a one way mirror has been not been installed at this center yet), she has a few questions about some of the reactions her child had to some of the activities. She is also curious about some of the changes in behavior from this week to three weeks ago during her daughter's first session. The therapist answers all her questions and they briefly discuss their expectations for the following weeks. They open the door and mother and daughter reunite. They hold hands, waving goodbye as they exit the lobby. The therapist waves goodbye, and takes a few minutes to rest and prepare for her next case.

Session B:

A small girl with shiny black hair pulled back into a ponytail fastened by a rubber band with the cartoonish face of a green frog attached enters the room. She takes a second to adjust her skinny pink hair band and push her bangs back under them. She enters the empty room tentatively but with enough curiosity to glance around for hints as to what today's games might be. Still holding her therapist's hand, she takes a quick glance at the mirror on the wall to her left. She knows Mom is waiting in that room, and that this other lady that she plays

> with every Wednesday is nice enough. This is not the first session, so the girl is not too scared. She recognizes the fun lady she played with last week. But she still seems unsure about why she is here or what she is supposed to do. She looks up at the lady for any indicator of what her afternoon will be like. The therapist, a middle-aged woman with short black hair cropped neatly into a bob that tapers at the neck, is dressed comfortably in black slacks and a loose button down shirt. The woman smiles reassuringly to her client, and welcomes her back to the center. They sit down and begin as the therapist notes all the healthy beautiful attributes of the girl, from the ten wiggly toes and fingers to the shiny brown eyes and jet black hair. Over the next 30 minutes, they move on to other activities, ranging from a hand-clapping activity like Sse-Sse-Sse to a cotton ball race (blowing a cotton ball across the room) and a makeshift basketball game using balled up newspapers. They wind down with a snack, as the therapist and the five-year old client take turns putting cone-shaped corn flavored chips on their fingers. They laugh at how silly their "nails" look and take turns eating the chips. The therapist also offers the little girl a small bottle of a sweet and tart yogurt drink, which she sips with gusto through the tiny straw. Together, they lean in closer, listening to the sound of the crunching noises and enjoying the last few moments of the session. Finally, they sing a song and close the session, holding hands and walking to the door. While another therapist watches the little girl, drawing pictures on a table in the lobby, the therapist and mother enter the room for a quick consultation. Because the mother was watching the session from the room next door, she has a few questions about some of the reactions her child had to some of the activities. She is also curious about some of the changes in behavior from this week to three weeks ago during her daughter's first session. The therapist answers all her questions and they briefly discuss their expectations for the following weeks. They open the door. Mother and daughter reunite, hold hands, and wave goodbye as they exit the lobby. The therapist waves goodbye, and takes a few minutes break before her next case.

The sketches of sessions I observed in the US or in Korea might be nearly the same in types of activities. For the most part, variation in activities and interaction were due to the type of case or the unique needs of the child, not dramatically different cultural paradigms.

Both of the therapists in these two sketches attended graduate school and had degrees in psychology, social work, and child development. They also went through the same training program to gain certification prior to these sessions. But there are also crucial differences. While the certification process may have been structurally the same, the therapists' experiences were also situated in contrasting paths of professional development. Therapists in the US most likely had a separate license in counseling, managed and regulated by her home state. This play therapy certification served as an additional specialty to supplement her practice. On the other hand, the therapist in Korea had no state structure to depend on (or report to) for regulation, standardization, and legitimization. Her "license" to practice was thus explicitly tied to this certification process.

Expert networks like the one at the center of this study span many countries and many structural variations. Meanwhile, the internal cohesiveness of a transnational training program for child psychotherapists assures continuity across cultures and locales. Because the majority of fieldwork was conducted in Seoul shadowing and interviewing therapists, the primary issues discussed in the preceding chapters can be thought of as locally specific and particular to Korea's governmental structure, history of policy development, and cultural perceptions about mental health. But in its particularity, Seoul lends itself to more transnational considerations. The psychotherapists in Korea who use elements of play to treat children with a variety of disorders, ranging from ADHD to depression, appear at the heart of this ethnography. Most of the therapists I worked with had been trained, at least partly, through workshops in the US. American trainers led these training and certification workshops. A small handful of practitioners were trained entirely in Korea, but even then, they had been greatly influenced by concepts and practices from abroad. This ethnography thus straddles the highly specific issues that guide and challenge the emergence of counseling and therapy for children in Korea, while fully acknowledging that this arena of contemporary Korean society and culture is also influenced by theories and practices circulating on a more global scale.

FIDELITY AND FLEXIBILITY

Extending these questions of translation to broader problems of adequation is important in terms of inquiring more broadly about "the action of bringing one's concepts in accord with reality, words with things, mind with matter" (Maurer 2005, xiii). In many ways, this precarious balance between fidelity and flexibility in transnational program adaptation mirrored my own dilemmas around translating the words of my interlocutors. Despite the fact that I had observed a more flexible approach to rethinking program adaptation as a form of cross-cultural translation, I did not allow this level of openness as I began my own endeavors. I had been conducting nearly every interview in Korean for several months while living in Seoul, painstakingly attempting to transcribe/translate them into English because I knew that I would be publishing in the latter language after fieldwork. Whenever uncertain, I would ask colleagues for their advice. Not all of them would agree with one another, and when they would respond with, "This is basically what they said: [insert translation]." At first, I interpreted "basically" as a kind of compromise—a substandard elementary translation for the meaning I wanted to capture from the speaker and relay to my readers. So I would reply with the earnestness of a young, slightly neurotic researcher, "But that's not *exactly* it. I need to be *precise*." One day, an interlocutor who had completed her own dissertation just a few years ago responded, "I understand. But you're not going to get any closer to the meaning if you go word for word like that. You have to go by what the person was saying in general." I nodded, thinking that I understood, and then proceeded to return to an excruciatingly slow process of translating my interviews, cross-referencing terms I was not certain of and still not understanding the depth of my interlocutor's words. Eventually, I began to note how often I encountered several key words that, no matter how many hours I labored or how many electronic dictionaries and experts I consulted, simply had no translation. I asked myself, "What do you do when there is no equivalent in sight—at least not one that is agreed upon by all?" It was then that I began to fully understand what my interlocutors meant by "basically" and "saying in general." They were not encouraging me to settle for loss of detail for the purpose of quick and easy translation but rather, they were encouraging me to let go of rigid compliance to equivalence in favor of a more meaningful commitment to adequation. Fidelity to the deeper meanings behind people's words did not hinge on word for word equivalence but rather, on reflections of intent to bring concepts in accordance with reality and words with things, thoughts, and feelings.

This is undoubtedly a common experience for many anthropologists, researchers, or any bilingual individual and I do not claim it as a special discovery. However, I note the mundane frustrations of fieldwork methodology here because it led to an unusual turn in this research. Words without equivalence soon became indicative of the flexible meanings and movements of play therapists. For example, maeum was a word that could signify both heart and mind, which proved to be an important ambiguity because it created a doubling term for therapists who advertised their services in treating cognitive and emotional disorders in children. In one word, they could evoke thinking *and* feeling. Treatment of the mind and treatment of the heart also allowed the therapists to position themselves close to psychiatry and the psychological sciences but evoke the kind of empathy of counseling for more emotional matters.

As I obsessed over preserving some sort of "fidelity" to my informants' words in my writings in English, and noted the sometimes productive meanings found in the failure to translate as I initially understood it, I also encountered a small handful of expatriate therapists through snowball sampling. These individuals were North Americans who had been living in Korea for several years, oftentimes over a decade. Some were close colleagues with Korean practitioners and others were independent practitioners that I found through online forums and websites. They spoke Korean with varying degrees of fluency, but conducted all of their sessions in English. For this reason, it was not surprising that most of their client-pools also consisted of expatriates living in Korea. I began to interview them, thinking that it would be useful to listen to other perspectives about trends in psychotherapy in Korea.

Several therapists noted that while most of their clients were English-speaking expatriates, several "Korean-Koreans" had also sought their services recently. At the time I was conducting research in Seoul, it was not uncommon for "Korean-Koreans" to be quasi-fluent to fluent in English, as many had been trained from an early age to master English for the sake of academic requirements and increasing future viability as a cosmopolitan citizen and a worker in a global marketplace. So I commented half-jokingly, "Maybe they just wanted to practice their English? Koreans around here speak English pretty well, or at least try to, especially the younger ones." And then I was struck with the oddity of the therapists' responses, "No, that's not it. Some of the ones that contacted me had a very hard time speaking English fluently." Why, then, would they go through the trouble of seeking out one of the few English-speaking therapists in Seoul when there were others that could converse with them in their native tongue?

Dr. Yim was one of the therapists I interviewed who recounted his experience treating clients who wanted to "do therapy" in English despite having difficulty speaking the language. A young therapist who works with both expatriates and locals, Dr. Yim told me how surprised he was when Koreans initially began to seek him out. Of the therapists from North America that I spoke to, Dr. Yim was most proficient in Korean, but still not comfortable enough to conduct full sessions in Korean. He thought that this would be a barrier given the limitations produced by language barriers, but his clients responded that they would actually *prefer* to do therapy with him in English rather than find a native Korean speaker. "Some Koreans have come in. Well, there are two things I noticed. One is that hierarchical language prevents a feeling of shared experience and feeling free when the language is formal. The second is that language barriers can allow for more creativity by expression through metaphors," remarked Dr. Yim. These points raised by the Korean clients were surprising to both Dr. Yim and myself because we had not considered that speaking in a second language in which one was less fluent could be preferable, particularly in situations where one was trying to master adequation and find words for thoughts and feelings that were already so difficult to do even in one's first language.

Three primary explanations for this phenomenon came to light during the course of my interviews. The first was that, by consulting an expatriate therapist, these clients were doubly assured that they would not run into any friends, colleagues, or neighbors. This assured them of bypassing any potential stigma associated with care for mental health issues. The second reason was that they felt they could avoid many of the constraints of speaking in their own language by speaking in English. Because English does not require a distinction between informal, formal, and honorific conjugations of verbs, they could escape the power differential that often separates two individuals varying in status (whether by age or by professional status and level of expertise). The words themselves could escape the power differential between therapist-client and doctor-patient while the themes might be afforded a more "open" interpretation than clients felt they could receive in Korean settings where they would be constrained by their own sense of cultural appropriateness. Finally, Dr. Yim alluded to the productive possibilities of limitations in language.

In many introductory cross-cultural psychology courses, lecturers often stress the helpfulness of cultural similarities between therapist and client. In reality, cultural similarities can both enhance and hinder treatment (Rodriguez et al. 2008). Language is less optional, as common sense would have us believe that too much difference would be a barrier to communication. This is a pragmatic and important consideration, especially in light of the advocacy efforts of many health educators who lobby for better translators and translated resources dealing with medical knowledge and care in immigrant communities. This push for better services also raises questions about the code of ethics for translators (Dysart-Gale 2005). But in this case, Dr. Yim began to speak of the productive possibilities of communication when words were insufficient and how this sometimes allowed more opportunities for breakthrough. In the absence of common linguistic ground, or someone to serve as a translator to find trans-linguistic equivalents, clients relied on metaphors, word pictures, and other devices to communicate emotions and experiences. They came to experience more freedom rather than more restriction through the process of conveying their feelings through new words and meanings.

In addition to finding meaning through metaphors and word pictures—things that others might initially see as last-resort measures for communication by a tourist on vacation rather than opportunities for breakthrough in conveying deeply personal moments of psychological turmoil—the clients also sought out an English speaking therapist in order to find common ground. This notion of common ground had to do with using English in place of Korean, which requires different conjugations for informal, polite, or honorific relationships. Korean is a language that not only communicates the substance of the message but also indicates the relationship between the speaker and listener. In her own research, anthropologist Dorinne K. Kondo notes some common experiences with Japanese speakers. Like Korean, Japanese is a language that depends on conjugation of verbs according to the relationship between speakers. Kondo notes that a person could not "utter a sentence without communicating at least two things: (1) the actual content of the message itself, the referential meaning; and (2) a metamessage about the relationship between the speaker and the listener, an indexical meaning"

(1987, 243). The message and the messengers are automatically contextual to the relationship and the situation in languages where expressions indicate "intimacy and distance, formality and informality" (245).

During our conversation, Dr. Yim and I talked about the power of switching languages and finding new meaning in second languages. Dr. Yim said that the three phrases—loan words—used by his Korean clients who said they would prefer to speak in English were "even playing field," "liberty," and "freedom." These were things they felt they could achieve by using English and in "Western-style" therapy. Less formal language, offered by English, allowed his clients to feel "more free" in disclosing their struggles to a therapist.[4] And when they felt the constraints on freedom due to lack of vocabulary, Dr. Yim found ways to allow his clients to communicate using simplified language that served as metaphors for how they felt about a more complex matter. He spoke of the power of "word pictures" and how "clients sometimes also bring in their own pictures, and even though it's really simple in terms of language, it can be powerful in conveying meaning."

Dr. Anderson was another young therapist, just slightly older than Dr. Yim, who reflected at length about his sessions with foreigners, kyopos (Korean-Americans), and locals (Korean-Koreans). I did not ask him about any specifics regarding cases, nor did he provide any information of that kind. He did, however, shed light on the kinds of dynamics that led to a less successful result than the Korean-Koreans who sought out Dr. Yim. Though his examples were of Korean-Koreans who might not like his "Western style" they also support Dr. Yim's contention that Koreans who seek less hierarchical or less directive counseling tend to prefer "therapy in English." Dr. Anderson mentioned one local who came to him for only one session. When the client did not return, Dr. Anderson wondered why he had discontinued. Admittedly, he said that this could be for a wide variety of reasons. For example, the problem might have resolved itself or the client could have come to the general conclusion that he did not really want counseling. Dr. Anderson suggested a third option, which was that he might not been directive enough to suit his client's tastes. Dr. Anderson contextualized this final statement, saying, "Actually, that's one common complaint among foreigners who go to Korean therapists (who speak English and sometimes offer to treat expatriates)—that they're too directive."

He then clarified the not-directive-enough vs. too-directive discussion with a story about an expatriate couple—a feminist and her husband—who went to a Korean therapist. "The therapists basically said, 'You need to be a good wife.' And the lady was not having that! Even the guy was kind of shocked, and just said, 'we just want to get along better' in response," said Dr. Anderson. In his stories, Dr. Anderson paints a picture of the opposite side of the coin to Dr. Yim's narrative. For Dr. Anderson, many expatriate clients found Korean therapists to be too directive. He then assumed that

Korean clients might find him too non-directive, and not return for his "Western-style" therapy.

In examining their reflections side by side, I suggest that people may seek or avoid different types of therapies, not based on what is more familiar to their linguistic or cultural upbringing, but rather by the kind of relationship they prefer and perceive as more conducive to working through a problem with a therapist. Some Koreans did in fact choose the more Westernized practitioner and type of therapy. In that style, they found a degree of freedom they felt they could not find with someone who spoke the same first language as themselves. When I asked Dr. Anderson to clarify why someone might have problems with being too directive, he replied that by doing so, the therapist could signify that "I'm the expert. There's no room for consultation and no room for discussion."

As I began to open up to the possibilities provided in spaces of limitation and the power of simplified stand-ins as metaphors for complex struggles, I began to realize that this is what the play therapists were also trying to accomplish. Although the kind of play therapy my interlocutors were practicing intentionally removed the emphasis on speech and shifted focus to the interactions achieved through play, they were still dealing with questions about adequation in expressing thoughts and feelings through play. Although they were mostly Korean women treating Korean families (locals to locals), they were gaining popularity in their communities and neighborhoods because play creates an "even playing field" where socio-emotional development could be attended to apart from hierarchical metrics often placed in the educational realm. It was not about a child's verbal prowess or their talent as a musician or artist, but simply about that carefree moment when mother and child enjoy the delight of one another's glance in a game of "Peek-a-Boo" or when two children blow puffs of air at their cotton balls as they race each other across the room. By using play, and simple childlike games and activities, child therapists in Korea were aiming to address the complexity of social interaction, which was a struggle for many of their young clients.

At one child counseling center, I asked two co-owners and therapists, "Is play therapy for cases when you can't do therapy verbally? For speech problems?" to which the first therapist replied, "No." Her colleague quickly clarified:

> To the extent that I'm dealing with something, I can express that verbally. Children who come to talk about that—many can verbally express themselves but for those that can't, like developmentally delayed children who might have difficulty expressing their problems, I use play instead. Therapeutic meaning is thus found through play. As children play and we communicate through interaction, we can figure out where this child is at.

In short, play was an active "word picture" and moving metaphor for complex concepts similar to the "word pictures" locals created in their sessions with expatriate therapists. Where speech created ruptures in the process of adequation, meaning was not lost. It was found.

A few days later after our interview, Dr. Yim emailed me an article that he had briefly discussed and summarized during our interview. In addition to being a therapist and conducting one-on-one sessions with both expatriates and locals, Dr. Yim also served as a consultant in cross-cultural training for expatriates. He had been reviewing the logistics of moving to a new country and adjusting to a new culture, when he began to also incorporate a discussion of words that had no direct translation (from Korean to English, French, Spanish, etc.). These were words like maeum and jeong.[5] The memo caught my eye because it replicated many of the concerns I had experienced in my own translation work as an anthropologist conducting fieldwork in Korean, knowing I would be writing and publishing in English. I was normally quite wary of any generalizations of differences between cultures (or clients) in cross-cultural psychology articles, but I found both authors to be refreshingly straightforward about their findings. Neither Dr. Yim nor the authors of the memo tried to oversimplify difference nor find exact translational matches for concepts. Instead, they spoke of words as conceptualizations of individuals' relationship to emotions and to others.

In the memo, Christopher K. Chung and Samson Cho introduced themselves as medical doctors at Harbor-UCLA Medical Center who were drawing from their work dealing with psychopathology among the Korean-American population in Los Angeles. Clearly, Korean-Americans are not stand-ins for Koreans when conducting research, but because they were working with a large immigrant population, I found the doctors to be considering some key issues of translation and communication. They wrote, "Before I introduce the concept of *jeong*, I would like to emphasize that this must not be considered as just a stereotype of Koreans or Asian populations. I would rather view these findings regarding the significance of *jeong* as very useful to understanding the nature of human emotions and its role in family and social structures" (Chung and Cho 2008). This struck me as an important and astute caveat provided by both authors from the beginning, as they attempted to elucidate culturally specific concepts without bundling together stereotypes so often produced by discussions of "culture-bound" syndromes like hwa-byung.[6] The memo also included a descriptions of jeong as having flexible meanings that incorporate both Japanese meanings such as jyo (nuances of sentimental feelings when used in conjunction with another word—nin-jyo) and Chinese meanings of the jeong character (aspects of loyalty and reciprocity in relationships).

Drs. Chung and Cho introduce the concept of jeong, not in terms of a comparative analysis of closest meaning to an original word, but rather as a way for Koreans to denote "location." Locational difference was a major point that Dr. Yim focused on during our interview. "*Jeong* seems located not only inside of our hearts but also outside. In other words, the location of *jeong* is between individuals. It can be difficult to understand an emotion as being seated outside of an individual's heart, yet it may be related to the idea of collective emotion," stated Chung and Cho.

Dr. Yim was using this memo for training North American and European therapists to pay attention to the "location" of feeling that they might have to adjust to when speaking with the Korean counterparts. He was teaching his colleagues to 1) pay attention to words that had no direct translation in English and 2) to pay attention to a shift in understanding self and relationships that was signified by the word itself. Rather than be frustrated at the lack of equivalence, Dr. Yim was pointing out how ruptures could be seen as opportunities to understand meaning and intent more deeply, rather than more superficially. Meanwhile, Korean locals were coming to Dr. Yim as clients precisely because of the relational aspect that the discussion of jeong referred to. Their ability to "do therapy" in English allowed them to depart from the hierarchy created at the power ridden nexus located between client and therapist and underscored by the verb conjugations they would have to use in Korean.

Play, too, created "an even playing field" upon which "freedom" could be experienced apart from the structured and sometimes stigmatized nature of traditional mental health options for children. Translation—or perhaps more accurately described as adequation—was happening at every scale and intersection: the child articulating their thoughts and feelings in the act of play; the therapist engaging in that conversation where play served as a mediational event between the two individuals; and for therapists in Korea and the US sharing knowledge and expertise as they co-created a therapeutic program that was simultaneously addressing fidelity *and* flexibility.

Play itself is defined by elements of spontaneity and flexibility. Play can happen during or through a game, which has defined rules and guidelines, but it does not need to adhere to the rules of the game. Play anticipates surprising results and calls on those who want to participate to be creative. The perfect play is, in fact, imperfect in that it does not follow precisely the set plan. Similarly, the perfect adaptation or translation of playful activities for children in therapeutic sessions is not about predetermined standards of perfection or equivalence. Where difficulties lie in finding equivalence, ruptures in adequation are experienced. But if we begin to see such ruptures as opportunities to produce deeper and more accurate descriptions of meaning, then the circulation of knowledge and practice takes on a whole new life.

Chapter Seven

What Play Proposes

> If "desire" in the psychoanalytic sense is proper only to human language—constituted subjects, then sensuous "joy" is what play-constituted beings experience. Like copresence, joy is something we taste, not something we know denotatively or use instrumentally. Play makes an opening. Play proposes...Play is not making a living; it discloses living. Time opens up.
> —Donna Haraway, *When Species Meet* (2008, 240)

Play is more than a game or collection of rules. One can certainly play by using the rules of a game. One might even find playful attributes within a game. But a game itself is not play. Play is the discovery of the delightful and the unexpected, found outside the lines of the predictable but within the boundaries of meaningful and caring interaction. For example, a bite on the arm may be delightful and unpredictable for one child but not for the child who screams in pain and surprise, wondering how playtime had gone awry. This would not be seen as a meaningful and caring interaction for the injured child.

There is a great hopefulness in play because it is based on the human spirit rather than material resources. A cardboard box can be a rocket ship, and popping soap bubbles can be just as powerful a way of connecting with others as a trendy doll or a complicated game.

As parents and children in Korea were introduced to different types of play-based therapy, they began to think about the work of play. For the children being treated, play did not come easily. However, play was something through which they could grow, learn, and eventually do "effortlessly" as they engaged more and more with their family and peers. For parents interacting with their children inside and outside of therapeutic sessions, play became the medium through which they could connect with their children. In play, they were able to take hold of the hopeful promises of therapy without feeling the cumbersome socio-historical specter of stigmatized mental health services.

Meanwhile, a small group of women also began to reflect on the work of play and what that meant to their own professional development. They continued to reflect on their practices as they honed their skills in play therapy, reporting back to mentors in Korea while also becoming part of a transnational network of theory and practice. The translation of several play therapy programs from the US to Korea included a range of theoretical frameworks and a diverse set of strategies and skills. In some cases, this translation was seen more as a transfer of packaged content, from one locale to another. For others, translation was embraced more wholly as a means of engaging in a continuous refinement of theory and practice through co-produced knowledge. Co-produced knowledge emerged at the interstices of local and global, universal and particular, and program fidelity and flexibility.

Some, if not all, translation attempts experienced ruptures. Some ruptures were miniscule and, in the grand scheme of things, still looked fairly seamless to the outside observer. Other ruptures were moments where flows reverted to traditional top-down hierarchies that follow many of the dynamics one might expect in West-centered distribution of knowledge/power that demands "provinces" to conform to "core" norms. Others used those ruptures as opportunities to reflect on alternative—and more co-productive—modes of knowledge production that decentralized knowledge/power.

Rather than dismissing ruptures as barriers preventing me from getting to the real heart of my study, I started to understand them as *productive* gaps. The ruptures came to take on as much, if not more, meaning than the flow, the destination, and the final product. It was through these ruptures that meaning—whether reflecting deeply engrained ideas about self as norm or reflecting more collaborative philosophies—emerged.

Productive rupture does not always mean positive, and positive really depends on the subject position of the person evaluating the situation, much of which might be influenced by their own sense of cost-benefit. But I argue that rupture can indeed be productive in the sense of generating the articulation of underlying values and intent and creating space for reflection. Play and translation are both acts that create space for productive rupture. Translation, whether of words on a page to another page or of programs to another locale, actually resembles play. Both are the kind of endeavors that are at their best when structure morphs into spontaneous new meaning.

Play does not have to involve another person. Neither does translation. A child might find joy in playing with a cardboard box turned rocket or boat and imagine all sorts of delightful scenarios alone. Translation of text might be done for my own sense of satisfaction or enhanced understanding. But if we think more deeply about these scenes, one is never really alone and devoid of relationship in the act of play or in the act of translation. Materials came from somewhere and bear the fingerprints of others who shaped them before they arrived in our own hands to be shaped for revised objectives. When any object is reinterpreted and reshaped, it places two or more people into relationship with one another.

Furthermore, play and translation take on new meaning when placed in social context. As joyful as any of the activities described above might be for a single player, new meaning and spontaneous joy is discovered through copresence. This brings along a world of complexity but the payoff is often worth the while when new relationships are forged, and old ones are made stronger through negotiated interaction.

Translation itself is an exercise in finding accurate descriptions to continue the circulation of ideas. In its most commonplace form, translation is exemplified in an ethnographer's struggle to translate transcripts from one language used in the field to another used in publication. But translation also occurred in more subtle ways; from the translation of thoughts and feelings into speech or action in therapy sessions to the translation of activities between therapists in an international network of practitioners, translation became an attempt to find deeper meaning through circulation of information and experience. Instead of simply following along established structural guidelines, translation gave life to ideas and practices. The kind of "loss to fidelity" we often think of in program adaptation, translation, and circulation became reframed as a desire to find more meaning and deeper meaning through communication and spontaneous co-creation. When conceptualized in more flexible terms, translation became a great metaphorical companion for play. Program adaptation became less about following the rules of the game and more about following the guidelines enough to ensure a safe space for spontaneous joy and meaning to emerge. It became the work produced by play and the work that produces play.

This ethnography about the work of psychotherapy and the work done by therapists and clients is indeed a serious thing. I hope that I have treated it as such throughout the preceding chapters. But I hope to have explored the power of all the playfulness involved as well. As Donna Haraway writes, "Like copresence, joy is something we taste, not something we know denotatively or use instrumentally. Play makes an opening. Play proposes (2008, 240). The reason play is different from game is because of its capacity to produce joy, which strays from a kind of instrumental understanding and depends more on structure creating space to discover new proposals. I suggest that translation, too, is at its best and at its truest intent when it strays from denotative or instrumental demands and allows space to create an opening where a new proposal might emerge. Both play and translation do more than simply transfer content from one person to another or from one group to another; they ask that relationships between people, things or ideas be discovered afresh and anew each time. They see possibility in each iteration rather than expectation of repetition with no difference.

Reducing play and work to dichotomies takes away from the incredibly serious work that play does in our lives. It also sterilizes work, which is often given new life when play is interjected. By play, I do not mean farce but rather, the spontaneity of thinking and feeling brought on by its proposal. It opens up time and space for ideas to emerge, perhaps facilitated by planning and protocol but not limited by it. Play, for the cultural anthropologist, is not just about work-life balance and "off the clock" musings with friends made in the field (though it does not exclude those options). Play is the semi-structured interview. Play is the grant proposal, the literature review, and the prospectus as they open up to the ethnographic material. Play is all the work of engaging and living, of participating whilst observing, and of becoming interlocutor instead of neutral interviewer.

Where play and work meet lie fascinating hybrids of socio-cultural phenomena. In these borderlands, hybrids ranging from public/private to personal/professional and nature/culture begin to emerge. The most pronounced hybrid I noted in this research was the work/play dynamic, which appeared as the substance of this study as well as in its theoretical and methodological considerations. While a great deal of important theoretical work has been done on explicating the role of play in culture and society, little has been written on all the work of play. By this, I mean the work done by play and the work that goes into making play possible. So much more work by a wide variety of thinkers needs to be done to better understand play as it appears in social contexts. I have attempted to begin this conversation by highlighting how play takes on new stakes when it enters the conversation with the stakes of work, and specifically with therapeutic work.

THE BORROWED AND THE NEW

Throughout this ethnography, play has articulated itself though hybrid narratives of work/play. Work/play creates space for creativity even when there is standardization and adherence to protocol. The creativity embroiled in these processes of *work* is not as far from the creativity inherent to *play*. In fact, anthropologist Gregory Bateson (1972) once discussed the role of play in culture as an example of an experimental system par excellence because the creativity inherent to play allows for the reconfiguring of new meanings through repeated behaviors. A cultural analysis of play and play therapy requires an examination of both text and context and the implications of play with respect to "deep play." Play is simultaneously the complete freedom to be creative and the reiteration of embedded rules applied in new contexts.

In its most obvious form, the work/play hybrid appeared in this ethnography as the work of play in psychotherapeutic settings. In some ways, I find the spontaneous generation of new knowledge borrowed from the structural rules of the game and from the contributions of past players a similar kind of co-production. Even as I write this new ethnographic piece, I am in conversation with decades and decades of anthropologists, critical theorists, and scholars from many other disciplines. I borrow from them but I also make them new through use.

In closing, I now turn to some key theorizations about play and challenge how they might be rethought to incorporate the significance of work, not as a foil but as something that can be included *within* play. How might this interjection and intervention affect the "reading" of text/context in ethnographic practices writ large, a practice whereby social scientists find themselves in the precarious position of being beholden to adhering to certain methodological standards in collecting data, analyzing information, and representing real people, places, and phenomena while also remaining open to the possibility of the unexpected. The unexpected can arise throughout the course of work in the field as well as work in the representation of that field.

In this ethnography, I have discussed how this tenuous balancing act between standardization and innovation is not only permissible but *necessary* in order to allow circulation to continue. The balancing act is one that is crucial to understanding various hybrid forms. These hybrid forms range from nature/culture and personal/professional to normal/pathological and work/play. Therapists regulate their practices and plan for their sessions as a way of not only organizing their own individual experiences but also maintaining coherence with the organizations to which they belong. And yet, in all of these modes of adherence, change is inevitable *and* desirable. In this way, the circulation and translation of new ideas and practices both defies and relies upon the duality of rules and creativity, or to put it another way, of work and play.

Despite the dismissal of simple things as "child's play," it is interesting to note that there has been some important scholarship attempting to understand the significance of play. Helen B. Schwartzmann (1976), William Empson (1975), Roger Caillois (1961), and Brian Sutton-Smith (1997) have all described various notions of play. Sutton-Smith argued that play could be studied as a contrast between texts (descriptions of play) and contexts (social, psychological, or environmental correlation to play as an event); studies of play had been read as either text (in the early 1900s) or context (around the late 1950s) but Sutton-Smith called for investigations that looked at play in terms of both text and context. Clifford Geertz brings this coupling together through the concept of "deep play" (1973). In his description of a Balinese cockfight in *Interpretation of Cultures*, Geertz borrows the concept of "deep play" from philosopher Jeremy Bentham. Geertz writes, "By it he means play in which the stakes are so high that it is, from his utilitarian standpoint, irrational for men to engage in it at all" (432). Play does the work of letting seemingly hidden contexts surface while also doing the work of keeping them contained and diffuse through its very nature as "just play." Play defies itself and promotes itself in the same breath, always pulsating with the liveliness of social interaction if one only has the time and sensibility to listen to its rhythm.

Johan Huizinga (1955) called attention to the profound significance of play when he said, "In play there is something 'at play' which transcends the immediate needs of life and imparts meaning to the action. All play means something. If we call the active principle that makes up the essence of play, 'instinct', we explain nothing; if we call it 'mind' or 'will' we say too much. However we may regard it, the very fact that play has a meaning implies a non-materialistic quality in the nature of the thing itself" (1). Jacques Ehrmann later built on Huizinga's significant work and contribution to the study of play while also providing a thoughtful critique (1968). Ehrmann wanted to broaden the notion of play and warned against the tendency to define play always (and only) in opposition to work. He writes, "Play or seriousness. This alternative is sometimes treated as a dialectic: play and seriousness which, in turn, implies a whole series of others: gratuitousness and/or utility; play and/or work; play and/or everyday life; the imaginary and/or the real; etc" (32). In this structure of logic, Ehrman argues that reality and seriousness is always given primacy over secondary definitions of play. Because of this primacy, I think it is imperative to think about the kinds of hybrids that might exist when these supposed opposites are brought into contact with each other.

Object relations theorists like Melanie Klein, and D. W. Winnicott have discussed play in the context of relationships. Other important figures in developing psychological theories of play have included Erik Erikson and Jean Piaget. Neuroscientists like Jaak Panksepp have also made several key arguments regarding the brain's role in feeling joy and engaging in play (2004). These are just some of the extensive texts that describe their work and the history of the theorization of play. I do not pretend that this ethnography competes with any of those. Rather, I gesture to the many hands that have formed the books read, the pages turned, and the ideas churned that all bear their fingerprints as I sat alone in work/play with this ethnography. My relationship with these borrowed ideas produced new meanings as I engaged in the rules of the game of scholarship, worked on this study, and ultimately found a way to work/play with new concepts and data. My "new" ideas were always-already produced in social context. They are products of co-created knowledge generated through the relationships built through work/play in the field with interlocutors that included a group of hardworking and earnest women seeking to change the mental health options for children in Korea and the workforce options for their peers. Somewhere between the psychoanalysts, the developmental psychologists, the neurobiologists, and the social theorists, *play found a way to draw from all types of work.*

Play makes use of cardboard boxes, newspapers, cotton balls, and thin air as well as computers, musical toys, and battery-operated train sets. I hope that this ethnography has made a gesture to do the same. I have drawn from many disciplines and from a wide variety of data. As they converge and diverge, new information and new ways of thinking/feeling about topics like education, child mental health, family support services, transnational knowledge production, local/global conversations, and nature/nurture emerge.

I have not proven that all work is actually play, nor all play actually work. Work and play can be defined separately. But where the two meet, there are many opportunities to observe the dynamics of work/play and see what lives and thrives there. Life found in work/play is influenced by structure but not determined by it. In the same way, structural constraints like time, money, and access to resources affect the kind of actions available to an individual. But they do not determine action to the extent of closing off the possibility of innovation. For example, play therapists with limited access to legitimizing structures and resources associated with the state find alternative forms of legitimacy through transnational networks and private regulatory bodies.

For an ethnographer with limited funding, time, or access, there are basic constraints and structural factors that influence what can and cannot be gleaned. With unlimited access to resources, one might imagine a "more legitimate" study impenetrable to critique but there is never a perfect scenario in which real research about real life and real people takes place. This often generates frustration, and there are certainly some pragmatic "minimums" and "must haves" involved just as there is no perfect scene of therapy or parenting but this does not mean that anything is permissible to the point of endangerment. (Recall the earlier point about a child gleefully and surprisingly biting their playmate's arm. Play should go beyond the boundaries of simply following the rules of a game, but refrain from placing another in harm's way.) And yet, this sensitivity does not preclude us from appreciating the unexpectedness provided by play. Having to follow the rules of the scholarly game at times has been frustrating but through some experimentation with work/play strategies, I have found that structure does not have to stifle the possibility of studying the unexpected and remaining open to moments that catch even the most plan-oriented person off guard. Spontaneity can arise out of structure, and the two are not necessarily mutually exclusive.

MICRO AND MACRO LESSONS

The "scenes" I have included in this book may seem mundane and minute: the details of a child entering a therapy room for the first time, an anthropologist building relationships with interlocutors in the field, two therapists talking to each other about how their day went, and conference attendees sharing stories. But some of anthropology's greatest contributions as a discipline have been full of minutia that teases apart broader cultural assumptions and puts together lived experiences to form a more insightful picture about social beings. It is in this vein that I have applied an anthropological lens to the social context of play therapy implementation and adaptation in Korea.

From a hyperlocalized perspective, the treatment room is one way of applying a scale to the topic of play therapy in Korea. The scene of the treatment room can be dissected into many work/play hybrids that construct a broader sense of livelihood for its participants. For the therapist, work/play is defined predominantly by work. Throughout the session, the therapist is thinking about the skills she has learned and how they might apply for this particular child in this particular moment. Therapists often comment on the effort that goes into making a session successful. But this is not to say that there is an absence of play. In fact, the therapists will be the first to admit that there *is* joy in the session and that they have fun as well. The paradox then lies in the fact that therapists often feel that they have done the best "work" when they are able to "just play" with the child; this means that the child was able to play and enjoy their session, and the therapist felt this joy in the process.

For the child, the session of work/play is also defined mostly by work. Children who are able to play are not the ones referred to treatment. Individuals diagnosed with attachment disorders are treated using play therapy precisely because they do not engage with others easily. Play requires work on their part, especially when they may feel awkward or hesitate to respond in earlier sessions. But both members of the team must put in a great deal of work to achieve the full force of play. The artificial work of learned behavior is not purely artificial because "work" is always dependent upon tapping into the proclivities and embodied (neurobiological or social or otherwise) dispositions of individuals to play.

From a national or regional perspective, past and present statistics and reports about child mental health, education, and social welfare in Seoul or in Korea illustrate another scale. From a transnational perspective, therapists in dialogue with one another as they adapt programs across locales demonstrate yet another scale. Reading minutia across scales, and paying close attention to the articulations of desire and discontent as well as the lived experiences of therapists, children, and families allows us to see the world in a grain of sand—and the grains of sand (that is, lived experiences and realities) in a world of broader socio-cultural phenomena.

If all goes well, what was once a game of "cottonball soccer" orchestrated by the therapist and child blowing fluffy white pieces of cotton back and forth to one another becomes a spontaneous moment of laughter and merriment. The participation of both participants requires the following of basic rules, while also leaving room for the unexpected. The cotton ball tends to fly in unexpected directions and both players find themselves adjusting how hard or softly they blow depending on how the ball seems to fly on the floor. Simply telling a distracted child to blow a ball in a straight line or instructing a withdrawn child to be more active and lively is structure without spontaneity. But the interaction of two workers, child and therapist, allows for work to slowly morph into play. Ultimately, the child concludes treatment no longer having to work at playing. Work has become play. For the client, the transformation represents a more linear narrative from **work** to **work/play** and finally to **play**. The linear narrative structures the terms of progress for treatment. For the therapist who occasionally experiences play throughout the session in moments of success and breakthrough, however, the ending is always **work/play**. Work never drops out of the equation because they are always "at work," doing their jobs as trained therapists and making a living.

The simple answer to explain the child's end of treatment as pure play and the therapist's end as always work/play might be reduced to income and material reward. The therapist makes a living and earns a salary through the work they do during these sessions. But this is not always the case. In many instances, the Korean therapists I worked with did not receive direct financial compensation for their efforts. Many offered treatment as part of their practicum or early apprenticeship. Perhaps they were rewarded with the necessary hours of training to complete certification which then resulted in salary and eventually converted to material reward. However, I looked a bit deeper into this process because most of the play therapists in this study, even those who were already certified and more established, were not profiting greatly from providing treatment. In this case, it became important to ask whether they have other sources of income that allows them to enjoy work/play in treatment sessions without the burden of producing results for material reward. Did they believe that eventually the program would become popular enough to result in profit (expanding from the current state of mostly volunteered hours of service during the process of earning a doctorate or depending on government subsidies for work at community/social welfare centers)? Or, were there other motives at work/play, such as belief in the inherent value of helping children? These kinds of macro questions emerged from tracing the cotton soccer ball across the room and following a group of professionals across borders.

In placing these micro and macro lessons alongside one another, I glean deeper insights about the kinds of work/play that can happen in certain therapeutic settings. For the play therapist, there is a constant negotiation and oscillation between the various forms that the hybrid, work/play, can appear as. Therapists use a technique called "attunement" to feel moments of anxiety, tension, and joy so that they can better anticipate the interactions that occur during play therapy. Donna Haraway describes a phenomenon similar to attunement through the concept of "isopraxis" which French ethologist Jean-Claude Barrey described as the "unintentional movements" exhibited by riders and horses. The muscles of riders and horses become so attuned to one another that they begin to fire together; this is more than mere coordination between two animal beings because even unexpected movements (when something goes wrong, for example) are met with very little time lag by an adept "ingrained" response (229). What is an instinctive response is also one that has been cultivated by repeated interaction—not reducible to mere repetition of learned behavior but rather, through interaction that nurtures the ability to respond to that which is utterly unpredictable.

The event of mutual collaboration in work/play not only rewrites the narrative of the experience as **work/**play, **work/play**, or work/**play**, but it also reconstitutes each of the players during the activity. Work/play relationships never quite escape their historical contingency but in the spontaneity of interaction and the unpredictability of the moment of relating, actors are made anew. Some women become professional therapists and working experts. Some women become savvy mothers open to treatment and proactive in finding services as yet another condition of consumer savvy and home/family management. Others accept treatment and attempt to shrug off a history of stigma. Children become both focused and liberated through the work of play.

Work/play is therefore a creative matter, an engagement with things as they were and are while also making them new. This is the broader sense of the experiment, in non-laboratory terms. Creativity is not born from complete disruption and anarchy but rather, in the momentary ruptures and mistakes that allow the parties to produce new things. The proposal of play (and work/play) lies in the way an event anticipates or asks for the new to emerge. Even in acknowledging structured dispositions of the actors (human or not, adult or not, pathological or not), this conceptualization of work/play moves beyond deterministic narratives.

I could write an entire book simply reviewing and studying the theorization of play. But it would leave little room to underscore all of the work/play that both the therapists and I did during this time frame. For the purpose of this ethnography, I have reflected on a few elements of play as it intersects with psychotherapy, Korea, and working expertise in order to show how play is a concept situated within a complex web of people who have contrasting definitions of play and are affected in different ways by play. I also bring these theories of play up at the end of this ethnographic study because play is not just theory for the musings of academics, but part of the lived realities and contested domains of so many other people, from parents and children to therapists. Play has real stakes and beckons real actors. Play therapy calls into question not only how play is done or what play is but also asks how play affects us. What does play do to us? What does it do to our relations with others?

As pediatrician, psychoanalyst, and object-relations theorist D. W. Winnicott once described it, play "belongs to health: playing facilitates growth and therefore health; playing leads into group relationships; playing can be a form of communication in psychotherapy; and, lastly, psychoanalysis has been developed as a highly specialized form of playing in the service of communication with oneself and others" (56). The work that goes into being able to play for the patient receiving care, and the work put forth by the therapist who uses play to treat, are both part of the growth of a larger and more diverse pediatric mental health sector. The work of these therapists demonstrates that the work of play is always work/play.

Notes

1. HOW PLAY WORKS

1. All names are pseudonyms to preserve anonymity, unless otherwise noted. I have used the term "Dr." combined with a surname to reflect the conventions for addressing elders or any professional in Korea. Additionally, all of my interlocutors were either PhD recipients or in the process of receiving their doctorate. A few interviewees in this ethnography were also medical doctors. I use actual names for public figures, or when specific public events are known to be linked to a specific person.

2. Research for this book was conducted from 2005-2009. From July 2007 to July 2008, I conducted intensive field research with a group of women who generously shared their hopes, struggles, and changing roles within this emerging profession. Shadowing the therapists and interviewing them took me to workshops in the US and Korea as a participant, observer, and translator (sometimes all at once).

3. William Blake famously used the phrase "to see the world in a grain of sand" in his poem "Auguries of Innocence."

4. Although I have used pseudonyms for all of my interlocutors in this book, I refer to specific names of people who founded specific organizations in the US because this information was gathered from publicly available sources. The individuals who appear by their real names have already been tied to their roles as founders of specific associations and institutes.

5. Although I conducted this interview in Korean, Dr. Tanaka provided insights from her experiences in Korea, Japan, and the US.

2. BETWEEN STIGMA AND DEMAND

1. SBS and EBS are abbreviations for Seoul Broadcasting System and Educational Broadcasting System, respectively. SBS is a major network, similar to NBC, CBS, or ABC in the US. EBS is also a popular network, but state-operated and focuses on documentaries or educational programs.

2. The government introduced a series of reforms, beginning over 30 years ago when they attempted to equalize opportunities for education across socioeconomic classes. Robinson's study showed that the reforms were not successful in diminishing educational inequalities in the classroom.

3. Lee is using the McCune-Reischauer Romanization form; the Revised Romanization for the word is seonginbyeong.

4. Ironically, some studies have shown a link between depression and ADHD. For example, ADHD symptoms often coexist with those of other disorders ranging from ODD to depression (Cormier 2008). This challenges the assumption that ADHD and depression are so different that one should be socially acceptable and the other stigmatized.

3. ALTERNATIVE LEGITIMACY

1. The first three 5-Year Economic Development Plans occurred from 1962-1977.

2. Milton I. Roemer suggests that health services evolved through a series of phases. Prior to industrialization, health care was "bought and sold in a market" like any other commodity, but religious groups and charities intervened in the market by providing services for the poor. After industrialization, governments stepped in with another form of "market intervention" to preserve the productivity and livelihood of workers. And finally, "as doctors and other health care providers became more numerous, governments recognized the need for assuring their competence. Specified education became required for a license to practice—constituting one more strong intervention against free trade in the marketplace" (1989, 62). While this narrative of development may be true in many of the cases that Roemer studied, it is not a satisfactory one for Korea. If anything, religious organizations, community groups, or families all comprised the "private sphere" writ large. An individual's health was managed in the private sphere when no larger social infrastructure existed. Add to this, the pervasive stigma surrounding any kind of psychological ailment, and it is easy to understand why mental health services were either not spoken about in public or managed entirely within the private sphere.

3. The word used here was nodong, which can be translated as either work or labor. It was striking for the therapist to use this word, which more often appears in the context of workers in settings such as factories.

4. In terms of economic capital, or explicit monetary value, the people I interviewed ranged in income and salary. For one hour of work (oftentimes a 30 minute session with the child, followed by 15 minutes consultation with the parent, and some extra time for setting up and cleaning up), therapists could receive nothing if they were volunteering, a small amount (enough to curb transportation costs), a free lunch, reduced pay around $15, or up to the $30-60 range.

5. In *The Too-Good Wife* (2005), Amy Borovoy examines the dynamics of women's support groups formed in the early 1990s by utilizing codependency vocabulary from American popular psychology. In Japan, one's individual state of mental health arose in the context of redefining what it meant to be part of a family and part of a nation. Both individual and social development were deeply entangled in the origins of codependency discourse as it landed and circulated in Japan. In Borovoy's case of codependency in group therapy circles for women married to alcoholics, there is the inter-cultural issue of American psychotherapeutic vocabulary being integrated in Japan. Her ethnography shows how the practice of group therapy and the discourse around co-dependency were taken from Western roots but translated and reinterpreted into the contemporary Japanese context.

5. A GOOD-ENOUGH PROPOSAL

1. Margaret Mead famously introduced examples of societies where the roles and temperaments of women and men were far more varied than the naturalized notions of masculine and feminine work previously used (1935).

2. Transferring skills as part of the professionalization process for play therapists is different from the concept of "transference" in psychoanalysis. It is important to note here the

difference between transferring and transference, just as I mentioned early on in this ethnography the importance of understanding the difference between attachment-based therapies and therapies for Reactive Attachment Disorder. The latter is what led to confusion early on in my research when scholars outside of child development and child psychotherapy—where attachment is better understood in broader dyadic terms—misrecognized these therapists for therapists who specifically treat RAD, which has its own cluster of debates. Those debates are important to address, but they are not the work of my interlocutors nor are they the work of this ethnography.

6. DISRUPTIVE TRANSLATION

1. Given this understanding of translation, it may be useful to reflect on Jacques Derrida's reading of Edmund Husserl. Derrida argues that the question, "what is the historico-semantic relationship between genesis and structure in general?" is not merely asking about language and genesis. It is asking about "the unity of the historical ground on whose basis a transcendental reduction is possible and is motivated by itself" (1978, 167). Derrida's différance is important in rethinking the concept of translation and its related problem of adequation; différance displaces the transcendental signified from the center of structure such that there need not be a fixed origin point for interpreting and translating language. This challenges the primacy of speech and thought over writing. By disrupting the teleology of signifiers and referents, Derrida contests the idea that there are linear chains of finding adequate translations and representation, each somehow falling further from an imagined origin point.

2. Choy's argument draws from Ernest Laclau and Chantal Mouffe who define "articulation" in Hegemony and Socialist Strategy as "any practice establishing a relation among elements such that their identity is modified as a result of the articulatory practices" (Laclau and Mouffe 1985, 105). This definition of articulation joins together the question of how "workers" are produced while studying the "work" itself.

3. Jaak Panksepp suggests that "underlying neural systems are designed so that one cannot easily be his or her own social partner or play companion" (289). In this way, the senses (the material reality of skin, nerves, hormones, and neural circuitry) are inextricably woven together with experience and perception. Play is also social in cases where "joy" seems contagious; an individual smiles or laughs just by observing others experience joy. Perception (which involves the brain, the body, and the environment) co-writes the narrative of play along with the senses. What makes Panksepp such a compelling theorist and researcher of play is the attention to scientific rigor in behavioral and laboratory studies coupled with his acknowledgment of social and cultural influence. He contests past studies suggesting sex differences in play on the basis of science—a lack of persuasive data. In doing so, Panksepp's work in psychobiology hearkens back to earlier arguments (albeit through different means and methods) by Margaret Mead in her groundbreaking ethnographies of gender, personality, childhood and childrearing in *Growing Up in New Guinea* (1930) or *Sex and Temperament* (1935).

4. This is not always the case. Many others will no doubt attest to the added stress of communicating in a second language.

5. "Jeong is difficult to define. One Korean-English dictionary defines it as 'feeling, love, sentiment, passion, human nature, sympathy, heart.' Although it is complicated to introduce a clear definition of jeong, it seems to include all of the above as well as more basic feelings, such as attachment, bond, affection, or even bondage," write Drs. Chung and Cho.

6. The culture-bound syndrome, added to the fourth edition of the *Diagnostic and Statistical Manual* (DSM), is one way that psychologists have tried to address the problem of cultural context. But this neatly packed addendum can be problematic for several reasons. A culture-bound syndrome infers that all other syndromes are not of the cultural variety and can exist as supplements to universal conceptualization of psychological struggle. Adding "culture" to the manual thus produces an exclusionary paradigm that creates space for culture—but only as supplementary. Epidemiologist Robert Hahn argues that the culture-bound syndrome is often an easy way of marking phenomena that seem exotic to the observer who is trained in Western

medicine (1985). In a commentary published in *Culture, Medicine and Psychiatry*, Margaret Lock revisits some of Hahn's arguments, but in the context of debates about adding culture-bound syndromes to the then current version of the DSM-III. She describes the project of Western medicine's "monothetic classification, grounded in the logic of Arisotle" as akin to what "Edmund Leach calls 'butterfly-collecting'" (1987, 36).

Bibliography

Abelmann, Nancy
2003 The Melodrama of Mobility. Honolulu: University of Hawaii Press.
Abouzeid, Leila
1983[1989] The Year of the Elephant: A Moroccan Woman's Journey Toward Independence. Barbara Parmenter, trans. Elizabeth Warnock Fernea, introduction. Austin: University of Texas, Austin.
Amsden, Alice
1989 Asia's Next Giant: South Korea and Late Industrialization. New York: Oxford University Press.
Anagnost, Ann
2004 Corporeal Politics of Quality. Public Culture 16(2):189-208.
Anderson, Gerard F.
1989 Universal Health Care Coverage in Korea. Health Affairs, Summer 1989; 8(2): 24-34.
Abu-Lughod, Lila
1991 Writing Against Culture. *In* Recapturing Anthropology: Working in the Present. R.G. Fox, ed. Pp. 137-162. Santa Fe: School of American Research Press.
Armstrong, Charles K.
2002 Korean Society: Civil society, democracy and the state. New York: Routledge.
Association for Play Therapy
2013 Milestones. Electronic document, http://www.a4pt.org/ps.playtherapy.cfm?ID=1158, accessed May 11, 2013.
Association for Play Therapy
2013 About Play Therapy Overview. Electronic document, http://www.a4pt.org/ps.index.cfm?ID=2385, accessed May 11, 2013.
Bakhtin, Mikhail M.
1981 The Dialogic Imagination: Four Essays. Michael Holquist, ed. Austin: University of Texas Press.
Bateson, Gregory
1972 Steps to An Ecology of Mind. New York: Ballantine.
Bhabha, Homi K.
1994 The Location of Culture. London: Routledge.
Beck, Ulrich
1992 Risk Society: Towards a New Modernity. Newbury Park: Sage.
Borovoy, Amy
2005 The Too-Good Wife: Alcohol, Codependency, and the Politics of Nurturance in Postwar Japan. Berkeley: University of California Press.

Bowker, Geoffrey, and Susan Leigh
1999 Sorting Things Out: Classification and Its Consequences. MA: Massachusetts Institute of Technology Press.
Callois, Roger
2001 Man, Play, and Games. IL: University of Illinois Press.
Callon, Michel
2007 What Does It Mean to Say That Economics Is Performative? *In* Do Economists Make Markets? Donald MacKenzie, Fabian Muniesa, and Lucia Siu, eds. Princeton: Princeton University Press.
Canguilhem, Georges
1991[1943] The Normal and the Pathological. Carolyn R. Fawcett and Robert S. Cohen, trans. New York: Zone Books.
Castro, Felipe G., Manuel Barrera Jr. and Charles R. Martinez Jr.
2004 The cultural adaptation of prevention interventions: resolving tensions between fidelity and fit. Prevention Science 5(1): 41-5.
Chang, Kyung-Sup
1998 Risk Components of Compressed Modernity: South Korea as Complex Risk Society. Korea Journal 38(4):207-228.
Chang, Kyung-Sup
1999 Compressed modernity and its discontents: South Korean society in transition. Economy and Society 28(1):30-55.
Chang, Suk C., and Kwang-Iel Kim
1973 Psychiatry in South Korea. The American Journal of Psychiatry 130:667-669.
Cho, Sun-Mi, Hyun-Soo Kim, Hyun-Jung Kim, and Yun-Mi Shin
2007 Factors Influencing Perceptions of Need for and Decisions to Solicit Child Mental Health Services by Parents of 9-12 Year-Old Korean Children. Child Psychiatry Human Development 38(4):279-286.
Cho, Sun-Mi, Hyun-Soo Kim, Hyun-Jung Kim, and Yun-Mi Shin.
2008 Perceived Need and Use of Child Mental Health Services in Korea. Community Mental Health Journal 43(4) [Epub ahead of print]. Electronic document, http://www.springerlink.com/content/0010-3853, accessed September 27, 2008.
Choy, Timothy K.
2005 Articulated Knowledges: Environmental Forms of Universality's Demise. American Anthropologist 107(1):5-18.
Chung, Christopher K., and Samson Cho
2008 Significance of 'Jeong' in Korean Culture and Psychotherapy. Personal correspondence received electronically on May 12, 2008. Electronic document, http://www.prcp.org/publications/sig.pdf, accessed May 12, 2008.
Clifford, James, and George E. Marcus, eds.
1986 Writing Culture: The Poetics and Politics of Ethnography. Berkeley: University of California Press.
Coombe, Rosemary
1998 The Cultural Life of Intellectual Properties: Authorship, Appropriation, and the Law. USA: Duke University Press.
Cormier, Eileen
2008 Attention deficit/hyperactivity disorder: a review and update. Journal of Pediatric Nursing 23(5):345-57.
Derrida, Jacques
1978 "Genesis and Structure" and Phenomenology. *In* Writing and Difference. Alan Bass, trans. Pp.154-168. Chicago: University of Chicago Press.
Desjarlais, Robert
1997 Shelter Blues: Sanity and Selfhood Among the Homeless. Philadelphia: University of Pennsylvania Press.
Dysart-Gale, Deborah
2005 Community Models, Professionals and the work of medical interpreters. Health Communication 17(1):91-103.

Ehrmann, Jacques, Cathy Lewis and Phil Lewis
1968 Homo Ludens Revisited. Yale French Studies 41 (Game, Play, Literature):31-57.
Empson, William
1975 Seven Types of Ambiguity. USA: Vintage/Ebury (Random House).
Epstein, Steven
1995 The Construction of Lay Expertise: AIDS Activism and the Forging of Credibility in the Reform of Clinical Trials. Theme Issue, "Constructivist Perspectives on Medical Work: Medical Practices and Science and Technology Studies," Science, Technology, & Human Values 20(4):408-437.
Erikson, Erik H.
1963 Childhood and Society. New York: W.W. Norton & Company, Inc.
Escobar, Arturo
1995 Encountering Development: The Making and Unmaking of the Third World. Princeton: Princeton University Press.
Esping-Andersen, Gøsta
1990 The three worlds of welfare capitalism. Cambridge, UK: Polity Press.
Estroff, Sue E., William S. Lachicotte, Linda C. Illlingworth, and Anna Johnston
1991 Everybody's Got a Little Mental Illness: Accounts of Illness and Self among People with Severe, Persistent Mental Illnesses. Medical Anthropology Quarterly 5(4):331-369.
Fabian, Johannes
1983 Time and the Other: How Anthropology Makes Its Object. New York: Columbia University Press.
Falk Moore, Sally
1987 Explaining the Present: Theoretical Dilemmas in Processual Ethnography. American Ethnologist 14(4):727-736.
Ferguson, James
1994 The Anti-Politics Machine: "Development," Depoliticization and Bureaucratic Power in Lesotho. Minneapolis: University of Minnesota Press.
Flynn, Marilyn L., and Young-Soon Chung
1990 Health care Financing in Korea: Private Market Dilemmas for a Developing Nation. Journal of Public Health Policy, Summer, 1990; 11(2):238-253.
Fox, Dennis, and Isaac Prilleltensky, eds.
Critical Psychology: An Introduction. London: Sage Publications.
Fujimura, Joan H.
1992 Crafting Science: Standardized Packages, Boundary Objects, and "Translation." *In* Science as Practice and Culture. Andrew Pickering, ed. Pp. 168-214. Chicago: University of Chicago Press.
Gallagher, Eugene B.
1989 Sociological Studies of Third World Health and Health Care: Introduction. Journal of Health and Social Behavior 30(4):345-352.
Geertz, Clifford
1973 Interpretation of Cultures. New York: Basic Books.
Gieryn, Thomas F.
1983 Boundary-Work and the Demarcation of Science from Non-Science: Strains and Interests in Professional Ideologies of Scientists. American Sociological Review 48(6):781-795.
Goffman, Erving.
1986 Stigma: Notes on The Management of Spoiled Identity. New York: Simon & Schuster.
Greve, Henrich R.
1998 Managerial Cognition and the Mimetic adoption of Market Positions: What You See Is What You Do. Strategic Management Journal 19(10):967-988.
Hahn, Robert A.
1985 Culture-Bound Syndromes Unbound. *Soc. Sci. Med.* 21(2):165-171.
Hall, Stuart
1992 New Ethnicities. *In* "Race", Culture and Difference. James Donald, James, and Ali Rattansi, eds. Pp. 252-259. London: Sage.
Hannan, Michael T., Glenn R. Carroll, and Lázló Pólos

2003 The Organizational Niche. Sociological Theory 21(4):309-340.
Haraway, Donna
2008 When Species Meet. Minneapolis: University of Minnesota Press.
Holliday, Ian
2000 Productivist welfare capitalism: Social policy in East Asia. Political Studies 48: 706-723.
Huizinga, Johan
1938 Homo Ludens. Boston: Beacon Press.
Illouz, Eva.
1997 Consuming the Romantic Utopia: Love and the Cultural Contradictions of Capitalism. Berkeley: University of California Press.
Im, Sook-Bin, Jung-Lim Kim, Se-Jin Ju, Mi-Kyung Kwon, Ju-Hee Kim, Ji-Hyang Kwon, and So-Woo Lee.
2004 Development of Child and Adolescent Psychiatric Nursing Practice in Korea, 1980-2000. Journal of Child and Adolescent Psychiatric Nursing 17(2):56-65.
Jernberg, Ann M., and Phyllis M. Booth
2001 Theraplay: Helping Parents and Children Build Better Relationships Through Attachment-Based Play. San Francisco: Jossey Bass Publishers.
Joyce, Kelly A.
2008 Magnetic Appeal: MRI and the Myth of Transparency. Ithaca: Cornell University Press.
Kataoka, Sheryl H., Lily Zhang, and Kenneth B. Wells
2002 Unmet need for mental health care among U.S. children: variation by ethnicity and insurance status. American Journal of Psychiatry 159:1548-1555.
Keller, Evelyn Fox
1983 A Feeling for the Organism: The Life and Work of Barbara McClintock. San Francisco: W.H. Freeman and Company.
Kevles, Bettyann H.
1997 Naked to the Bone: Medical Imaging in the Twentieth Century. New Brunswick: Rutgers University Press.
Kim, Chang-gyu
2008 Doctors see increase in number of mental health cases. Joongang Ilbo, February 26, 2008. Electronic document, http://joongangdaily.joins.com/article/view.asp?aid=2886632 , accessed March 24, 2008.
Kim, Yoon-Kyung, and Sheena Nahm
2008 Cultural Considerations in Adapting and Implementing Play Therapy. International Journal of Play Therapy 17(1):66-77.
Kondo, Dorinne K.
1987 Creating an Ideal Self: Theories of Selfhood and Pedagogy at a Japanese Ethics Retreat. Ethos 15(3):241-272.
Kumpfer, Karol L., Methinin Pinyuchon, Ana Teixeira de Melo, and Henry O. Whiteside
2008 Cultural Adaptation Process for International Dissemination of the Strengthening Families Program. Evaluation & the Health Professions 31: 226-239.
Kwon, Soonman
2003 Healthcare financing reform and the new single payer system in the Republic of Korea: Social solidarity or efficiency? International Social Security Review 56(1/2003): 75-94.
Kwon, Soonman, and Ian Holliday
2007 The Korean welfare state: a paradox of expansion in an era of globalization and economic crisis. International Journal of Social Welfare 16:242-248.
Kwon, Soonman, and Michael R. Reich
2005 The Changing Process and Politics of Health Policy in Korea. Journal of Health Politics, Policy and Law 30(6):1003-1025.
Laclau, Ernest, and Chantal Mouffe
1985 Hegemony and Socialist Strategy. London: Verso.
Latour, Bruno
1999 Pandora's Hope: Essays on the Reality of Science Studies. Cambridge: Harvard University Press.
Lave, Jean

1982 A Comparative Approach to Educational Forms and Learning Processes. Anthropology Education Quarterly 13(2):181-187.
Lave, Jean
1977 Cognitive Consequences of Traditional Apprenticeship Training in West Africa. Anthropology Education Quarterly 8(3):177-180.
Lave, Jean, and Etienne Wegner
1991 Situated Learning: Legitimate Peripheral Participation. New York: Cambridge University Press.
Lee, June J.H.
2001 Discourses of Illness, Meanings of Modernity: A gendered Construction of *Sŏnginbyŏng*. *In* Under Construction: The Gendering of Modernity, Class, and Consumption in the Republic of Korea. Laurel Kendall, ed. Pp. 55-78. Honolulu: University of Hawaii Press.
Lee, Sook Jong, and Kevin Hewison
2010 Introduction: South Korea and the Antinomies of Neo-Liberal Globalisation. *Journal of Contemporary Asia* 40(2):181-187.
Link, Bruce G., and Jo C. Phelan
2001 Conceptualizing Stigma. Annual Review of Sociology 27:363-385.
Liu, Lydia
1995 Translingual Practice: Literature, National Culture, and Translated Modernity. Stanford: Stanford University Press.
Lock, Margaret
1987 DSM-III as a Culture-bound Construct: Commentary on Culture-Bound Syndromes and International Disease Classifications. Culture, Medicine and Psychiatry 11:35-42.
Luhrmann, Tanya M.
2001 Of Two Minds: An Anthropologist Looks at American Psychiatry. New York: Vintage.
Matthews, John
1995 High-Technology Industrialisation in East Asia: The Case of the Semiconductor Industry in Taiwan and Korea. Tapei: Chung-Hua Institution for Economic Research.
Maurer, Bill
2005 Mutual Life, Limited. New Jersey: Princeton University Press.
Mead, Margaret
1930 Growing Up in New Guinea. New York: Morrow.
Mead, Margaret
1935 Sex and Temperament. New York: Morrow.
Ministry of Health and Welfare
2002 Ministry of Health and Welfare Report. Seoul: Ministry of Health and Welfare.
Mitchell, Stephen A., and Margaret J. Black
1995 Freud and Beyond. USA: Harper Collins.
National Health Insurance Corporation
2001 National Health Insurance Program in Korea 2001. Seoul: NHIC. Electronic document, http://unpan1.un.org/intradoc/groups/public/documents/APCITY/UNPAN009456.pdf (United Nations Online Network in Public Administration and Finance), accessed March 23, 2008.
Nelson, Laura
2000 Measured Excess. New York: Columbia University Press.
Nightingale, David, and Tor Neilands
1997 Understanding and Practicing Critical Psychology. *In* Critical Psychology: an introduction. Dennis Fox and Isaac Prilleltensky, eds. Pp. 68-84. London: Sage Publications.
Nuyens, Yvo, and Mary Ann D. Lansang
2006 Knowledge translation: Linking the past to the future. Bulletin of the World Health Organization 84(8):590-591.
Ortner, Sherry B.
1972 Is Female to Male as Nature Is to Culture? *Feminist Studies* 1(2):5-31.
Panksepp, Jaak
1998 The Quest for Long-Term Health and Happiness: To Play or Not to Play, That is the Question. Psychological Inquiry 9(1):56-66.

Panksepp, Jaak
2004 Affective Neuroscience. USA: Oxford University Press.
Park Jae Hyun, Suk Joon Yoon, Hye Young Lee, Hye Sook Cho, Jin Young Lee, Sang Joon Eun, Jong Hyuk Park, Yoon Kim, Yong Ik Kim, and Young Soo Shin
2006 Estimating the burden of psychiatric disorder in Korea (article in Korean). Journal of Preventative Medicine and Public Health 39(1):39-45.
Park, Jong-Ik, and Yong Sik Kim
2006 Changing needs and new perspectives for psychiatry and mental health services in Korea (article in Japanese). Seishin Shinkeigaku Zasshi (Journal of Psychiatry and Neurology) 108(11):1159-66.
Park, So Jin and Nancy Abelmann
2004 Class and Cosmopolitan Striving: Mothers' Management of English Education in South Korea. Anthropological Quarterly 77(4):645-672.
Park, Soo-mee
2007 The illness that dares not speak its name. Joongang Ilbo, February 22, 2007. Electronic document, http://joongangdaily.joins.com/article/view.asp?aid=2872653 , accessed January 17, 2008.
Parker, Ian
1997 Discursive Psychology. *In* Critical Psychology: an introduction. Dennis Fox and Isaac Prilleltensky, eds. Pp. 284-298. London: Sage Publications.
Prior, Margot, Shanya Virasinghe, and Diana Smart
2005 Behavioural problems in Sri Lankan schoolchildren: associations with socio-economic status, age, gender, academic progress, ethnicity and religion. Social Psychiatry and Psychiatric Epidemiology 40:654-662.
Resnikow, Ken, Tom Baranowski, Jasjit S. Ahulwali, and Ronald L. Braithwaite
1999 Cultural sensitivity in public health: defined and demystified. Ethnicity and Disease 9(1):10-21.
Rhi, Bou-Young
1998 Hundred Years' Psychiatry in Korea (article in Korean). Uisahak (Korean Journal of Medical History) 8(2):157-168.
Robinson, James
1994 Social Status and Academic Success in South Korea. Comparative Education Review 38(4):506-630.
Rodriguez, Carolyn I., Deborah L. Cabaniss, Melissa R. Arbuckle, and Maria A. Oquendo
2008 The role of culture in psychodynamic psychotherapy: parallel process resulting from cultural similarities between patient and therapist. American Journal of Psychiatry 165(11):1401-6.
Roemer, Milton I.
1989 National Health Systems as Market Interventions. Journal of Public Health Policy 10(1):62-77.
Rose, Nikolas
1998 Inventing Our Selves: Psychology, Power, and Personhood. Cambridge: Cambridge University Press.
Sakai, Naoki
1997 Translation and Subjectivity: On "Japan" and Cultural Nationalism. Minneapolis: University of Minnesota Press.
Schwartzman, Helen B.
1976 The Anthropological Study of Children's Play. Annual Review of Anthropology 5: 289-328.
Scofield, David
2004 Korean 'well-being' slogan for some, not others. Asia Times Online, October 20, 2004. Electronic document, http://www.atimes.com/atimes/Korea/FJ20Dg01.html , accessed April 10, 2009.
Seth, Michael J.
2002 Education Fever: Society, Politics, and the Pursuit of Schooling in South Korea. Honolulu: University of Hawaii Press.

Shin, Sun-Kyung, and Ellen P. Lukens.
2002 Effects of Psychoeducation for Korean Americans with Mental Illness. Psychiatric Services 53:1125-1131.
Sussman, Steve, Jennifer B. Unger and Lawrence A. Palinkas.
2008 Country Prototypes and Translation of Health Programs. Evaluation & the Health Professions 31:110-123.
Sutton-Smith, Brian
2001 The Ambiguity of Play. USA: Harvard University Press.
The Korea Daily
2008 Choi suicide sparks debate about Internet slander (article in Korean). The Korea Daily, Los Angeles edition, October 4: A1.
Theraplay Institute
2009 What is Theraplay? Electronic document, http://www.theraplay.org , accessed December 12, 2009.
Theraplay Institute
2013 About TTI-Who We are-Our Founder. Electronic document, http://www.theraplay.org/index.php/about-tti/who-we-are/our-founder , accessed May 11, 2013.
Traweek, Sharon
1999 Pilgrim's Progress: Male Tales Told during a Life in Physics. *In* The Science Studies Reader. Mario Biagioli, ed. Pp. 525-542. New York: Routledge.
Tsing, Anna Lowenhaupt
2000 The Global Situation. Cultural Anthropology 15(3):327-360.
Tsing, Anna Lowenhaupt
2005 Friction: An Ethnography of Global Connection. Princeton: Princeton University Press.
Walker, Janet S., Daniel Coleman, Junghee Lee, Peter N. Squire, and Barbara J. Friesen
2008 Children's Stigmatization of Childhood Depression and ADHD: Magnitude and Demographic Variation in a National Sample. Journal of American Academic Child Adolescent Psychiatry 47(8):912-920.
Weaver, Thomas
2009 The Ecology of Globalization; the Wolf at the Global Door. Bronislaw Malinowski Lecture presented at the Society for Applied Anthropology Awards Dinner, Santa Fe, March 20.
White, Leroy, and Ann Taket
1994 The Death of the Expert. The Journal of the Operational Research Society 45(7):733-748.
Winnicott, Donald W.
1971 Playing and Reality. New York: Routledge Classics.
Yi, Whan-woo
2013 Choi Jin-sil tragedy relived. Korea Times, January 8, 2013 Electronic document,
http://www.koreatimes.co.kr/www/news/nation/2013/01/116_128395.html , accessed January 8, 2013.
Yoo, Han Ik, Soo Churl Cho, Boong-Nyun Kim, Min Sup Shim, and Kang-E Hong
2005 Psychiatric Morbidity of Second and Third Grade Primary School Children in Korea. Child Psychiatry and Human Development 36(2):215-225.

Index

About the Author

Sheena Nahm, PhD, MPH, graduated from the University of Pennsylvania with a BA, double majoring in biological basis of behavior and anthropology. She went on to receive her MPH from Drexel University and her PhD in anthropology from UC Irvine. Dr. Nahm is currently director of a family engagement program at Para Los Niños, a nonprofit organization based in Los Angeles. In this role, she collaborates with schools, community residents, and parents to develop, implement, and evaluate sustainable strategies for transforming neighborhoods so that children and families can succeed in school and in life. Prior to joining Para Los Niños, Dr. Nahm worked in policy, communication, research and evaluation for various nonprofit organizations and educational institutions in Los Angeles, Philadelphia, and abroad. She has also taught at several colleges in the US, including The New School where she currently teaches courses in anthropology and sociology.

CPSIA information can be obtained at www.ICGtesting.com
Printed in the USA
BVOW07*1033141213

338971BV00004BA/6/P